EMBRACING THE SHADOWS

Navigating a Family's Mental Illness

Marlene Dunham

EMBRACING THE SHADOWS:
NAVIGATING A FAMILY'S MENTAL ILLNESS
By Marlene Dunham
© 2023

ISBN: 979-8-9895075-0-4

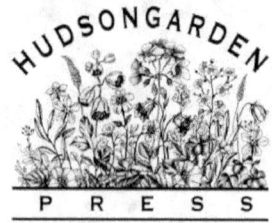

HudsonGarden Press

Photo Credits:
Lorraine Series © Stacey Halper 1993
Family Photos from the Halper photo archives

Typesetting and Cover Design:
Diana Ani Stokely

Dedication

To my three precious girls,

Allison, Melinda, and Elizabeth

You are the shining stars of my life.

Thank you for always supporting and encouraging my writing journey.

Through these pages, I hope to reveal more of myself to you, to share the depths of my heart and soul.

May these words offer you a deeper understanding of who I am and the immense love I hold for each of you.

MARLENE DUNHAM

Table of Contents

Introduction: Why Not Me?

This question has plagued me for years. It's been the unspoken punchline of many a conversation about my family history: Suspended in midair like that final silk thread from a spinneret.

Hanging fragile and vulnerable.

My comeback, always: "But I'm fine," and we all would laugh. The conversation would move on, But I would always wonder why. Why not—me?

This picture saddens me, as I see in it such hope. Children with great potential, prospects, and a future yet unmarred. I am saddened because I know the outcome. There would be two more children to come, and one, the youngest, would never have the opportunity to meet two of her siblings pictured here. That's little me, smiling on the left, 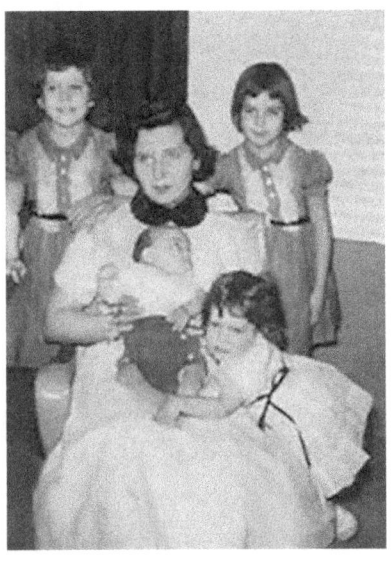 unaware of what the future holds. Lorraine is there on the right. Mom (Joan) is holding Warren, the baby, and Claudia is leaning on her lap. My dad, Burt, took the family photo.

I didn't fully recognize my family situation for many years. Like all small children, I perceived my life as typical. Of course, it was the only family life I had known.

I used to think I had a perfectly normal childhood growing up in an upper-middle-class family in a very good neighborhood of the Northwest Bronx. Still, all is not always as it seems.

We lived in Hudson Gardens, a giant of a building high up on a hill, overlooking Henry Hudson Parkway, in Riverdale, which was the northernmost point of New York City.

Urban legend tells of the eccentric Spanish Count Alfred De Silva, who built this edifice to resemble a Spanish castle in the early 1900s for his bride. It was built high enough to tower over all other structures with a clear view of the Hudson River, which he referred to as the castle's moat. The legend further reveals that the Count would use hallucinatory drugs, and on one occasion, when he thought he could fly, he fell to his death from his penthouse terrace. When our family lived there, my father told the story of watching Eleanor Roosevelt pull up in a limousine to visit some famous New York politician who now resided in that same penthouse apartment. It was quite a stately piece of architecture, complete with gargoyles and a uniformed doorman. As kids, of course, we would find the scariest places in this old stone building to explore and play. There were a lot of long dark hallways under the lobby between the storage rooms and the laundry room.

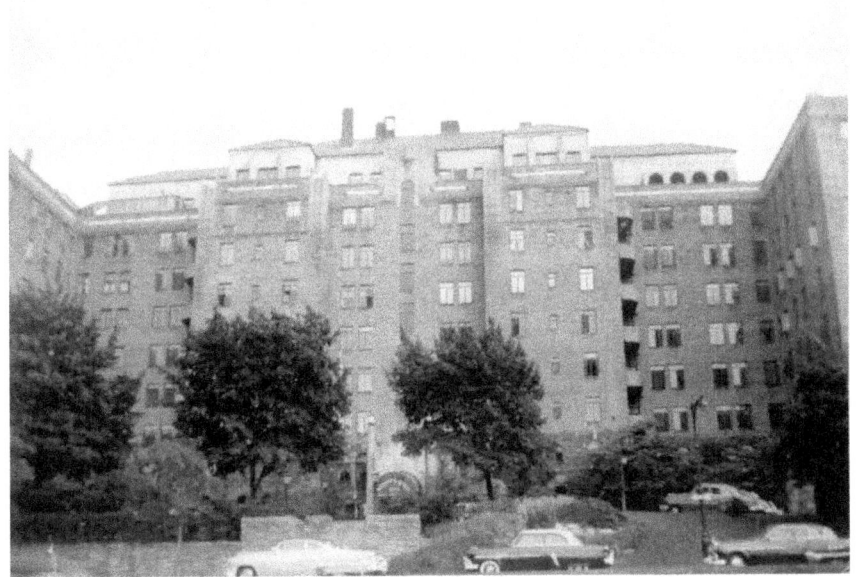

Hudson Gardens, Henry Hudson Parkway, 1953

We lived on the top floor just below the penthouse and one staircase below the roof. Tar Beach, we called it, as did every other New Yorker with a rooftop accessible to sunbathe. One summer, I got sun poisoning by laying on a towel spread over the black tar. Apparently, the tar attracted a lot more of the sun than sand does. Who knew? The next morning, I couldn't open my eyes.

Mom grew tomatoes on the roof, and Dad would spend hours with his sixteen-millimeter camera and tripod, taking pictures of sunsets that he would eventually splice together so it looked as if you were watching the sun setting on steroids. Seven seconds, and it was dark. The sunsets were spectacular. I later discovered the reason was because of all the pollution in the air. But there was nothing like a sunset over the Hudson.

On a clear night, you could see all the lights of the city. The George Washington Bridge, only five miles away, was always in sight from my bedroom window, except for the blackout of 1965. I remember looking out that window some nights at three or four in the morning and wondering where everyone was going. I would make up stories about their lives and the adventures they were having. The Parkway turned into the West Side Highway just a few miles south of my window. Frank Sinatra would give it the moniker "The City That Never Sleeps" twenty or so years later. I could attest to that right there from my bedroom vantage point, watching cars come and go to and from the city at all hours of the day and night.

Riverdalians, including my mother, did not like to associate themselves with the Bronx. Even to this day, when I tell people I am from the Bronx, I have to clarify that statement with "not the Bronx you see on TV." She would always insist we tell people that we lived in Riverdale.

The neighborhood was a mix of Italian and Irish Catholics and Jews. The only Black woman I ever knew as a child was Rebecca. She was our maid. It was the 1950s, and we fit right in. My mother was of Italian Catholic descent, and my father was Jewish.

The Kennedys lived in Riverdale for a few years in the late 1920s. More recently, some well-known residents included Carly Simon and her parents of Simon & Schuster fame. Steven Tyler grew up in Riverdale. And because of its proximity to Manhattan, many of the rich and famous lived there for periods of time: Ella

Fitzgerald, Lou Gehrig, Willie Mays, Tony Bennett, to name a few.

As in most neighborhoods in the 1950s and early 1960s, there was always someone to play with. There were 120 apartments in our building, with dozens of kids within a ten-year age range. The older kids we called the big kids. I think I reached big kid status at around nine or ten years old. Even though we were in the Bronx, we were surrounded by forest and spent many hours playing cowboys and Indians or setting up house among the trees. I distinctly remember sweeping dirt to make a flat surface for our humble abode and bringing items from our own kitchens to decorate. I don't know if this was with our parents' permission or even their knowledge.

We played Ring-a-levio, which is basically a game of tag, said to have originated in the streets of New York City. The rules are simple. There are two sides with the same number of players. There are two jails. There is one objective. Catch someone on the other team and put them in jail. Since we played in the back parking lot of the building, jail was always a car. The hood, the trunk, wherever. We also called it War on Cars. Those poor cars! Inevitably a resident would come out and yell at us to get off their car.

There was a massive staircase descending from the entrance down to the Parkway. When it was time for our First Communion, we Catholic girls would put on our white dresses and white veils like little brides of Christ. Along with the boys in their suits and ties, we would play 'wedding' on top of those steps. I remember 'marrying' Michael when I was about eight years old. We must have been first or second-graders, because that is when the Catholic Church considered us to be at the age of reason. (That is debatable.)

There were no cell phones. No supervision. "Just be back by suppertime" was our directive on our way out the door. We survived.

Times have changed.

PART 1 - THE FAMILY BEGINS

MARLENE DUNHAM

Joan and Burt (Mom and Dad)

My Catholic Italian grandfather and German grandmother were quite upset about my parents' marriage in 1947. They did not attend the wedding. My Jewish grandfather, on the other hand, was ecstatic. He had a son who, at twenty years of age, suffered at least one major mental breakdown, and they needed a nice, stable girl to take the responsibility out of their hands. It didn't even matter that she was a *shiksa*.

My mother was an only child of older parents. Her mother was overly protective and rather emotionless. She saw this as the opportunity of a lifetime, at eighteen years old and in love with this very handsome man. The fact that his parents were very well-to-do only encouraged her.

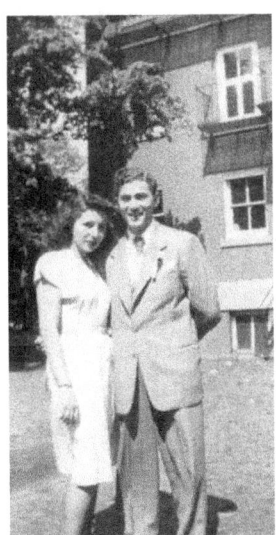

They met when she was only sixteen. He was a soda jerk at the local drug store, two and a half years her senior. Whenever she would come in and sit at the counter, he would come up with some strange concoction to offer. One she remembered was limeade with coffee ice cream. (Maybe that should have been a red flag!)

Joan and Burt, Bryant College, 1947

Mom graduated from White Plains High School the year she was sixteen and was on her way to Bryant College in Providence to take a one-year business course.

13

They dated throughout that year. He would go to Rhode Island to visit, and she would come home to White Plains every few months.

She was aware that he was seeing a psychiatrist, though not fully cognizant of his mental state, and could hardly fathom what life held in store for her.

He had his first breakdown after being discharged from the Army. He joined in 1944, towards the end of World War II, at eighteen years old. He was out less than a year later. Dad's story was that there was a leak in his gas mask, which caused lung problems, for which he received an honorable discharge along with VA benefits for the rest of his life. Mom and I felt that the discharge was probably due to a mental breakdown rather than lung problems. Having started smoking at age twelve, Dad smoked four packs of cigarettes a day for the next fifty years. His doctor encouraged him to continue smoking. It would keep him calm and perhaps stave off another episode. Just as the doctors told my mother to keep smoking during all her pregnancies, it would keep her weight down. It was the 1950s, after all. It may be hard to imagine smoking four packs of cigarettes a day (Chesterfield unfiltered) but let me tell you that the smell of cigarette smoke is entwined with almost every childhood memory I have.

Later, it would be the smell of cigarettes and lithium permeating his clothing, his apartment, his car. That will always be the smell of Dad.

It would not be unusual to open the freezer in our apartment to get some ice cubes out of that silver metal tray, only to see a long piece of cigarette ash lying on top. It was some sort of sport with Dad to see how long an ash could get before dropping — dropping wherever he happened to be. I was told he would smoke in the shower, with his arm hanging out the curtain so as not to soak the cigarette.

In the end, Dad died of heart failure, which was most likely caused by his smoking habits, but I do question the story of his Army discharge due to lung problems.

Mom went to visit her fiancé's psychiatrist in the days before the wedding. She was given the advice, "Run—run in the other direction as fast as you can."

Yes, by his psychiatrist! This seems most unprofessional, even for the late 1940s, but this is Mom's memory.

When telling her future father-in-law of the psychiatrist's warning, his response was something to the effect of, "Psychiatrists are all crazy themselves, so don't pay any attention."

She didn't. The lure of getting out of her home and marrying into a rich New York family was too enticing.

Dad was a salesman. He was an excellent salesman. I always said he could sell ice to the Eskimos. He certainly sold my mother on taking a chance on him, this good-looking, stylish man from a wealthy family.

I was aware each time my dad made an extended stay at the hospital. He went to a variety of hospitals, I would later find out: the good, the bad, and the downright ugly, depending on the length of the mania and level of his financial successes just before the depressive stage would knock the wind out of him and leave him gasping for air.

I was also aware that about three years after that photograph shown in the Introduction was taken, the baby in my mother's arms would go to live someplace else with people who could take care of him. Why couldn't we take care of him?

It would be a while, however, before I would connect the pieces to the puzzle that was my family and ask the question: Why not me?

Stomach Problems

One of my most vivid early childhood memories was of Dad standing on the threshold of our apartment door, Hudson Gardens, 65B, on a cold winter morning. My little bare feet were chilled by the linoleum. I was about six years old, and he was returning home from the hospital where he'd been for months. It seemed like an eternity for six-year-old me to be without my dad. I suppose this was Mom's first actual trial by fire—home alone with four children, ages one, two, six, and seven. I can only assume that her rich in-laws were paying the bills. They owed her that much, at least.

I remember being so relieved that he was finally home but, at the same time, anxious and uncertain because of the way he looked. I didn't really know where he had been and why. Mom said he was in the hospital because he had stomach problems.

With his wrinkled trousers and disheveled shirt, it looked like perhaps he had been wandering the streets of New York for the past couple of months. Dad was usually very well dressed and groomed, always smelling of English Leather, combined with the ever-present cigarette smell, of course. He had a red velvet smoking jacket he loved to put on in the evenings when he and Mom had friends over for drinks, though I don't remember Dad ever having more than a glass of champagne on New Year's Eve or a Dubonnet Cocktail during an important celebration. Dad was not a drinker, but he was always the life of the party. He was a sesquipedalian, a lover of big words. (And yes, I had to look that up.) Most of my parents' friends were my mother's, but he could always be counted on to be entertaining. He had a habit of arguing topics he may or may not know much about. Mom would drink her scotch, and Dad would pontificate.

One of his favorite phrases, which I must have heard dozens of times while growing up, was: "perched on the pinnacle of his own conceit." I never did figure out if he was talking about himself; although, to quote from a story he wrote called *Looking Good*, Dad says, "I was the epitome of sartorial splendor when I approached a prospective customer ..." I guess the reader must come to their own conclusion.

This man at the door that morning looked more like a homeless vagabond.

He had a full-grown beard, which was wiry and unkempt. I'd never seen my dad with a beard before, so it was a little disconcerting. His hair was knotted and dirty. But he was home. He'd gone to the hospital because of a stomach problem. At least now he was all better. But I wondered. Was he?

The year was 1956, and four of his six children were already born. Lorraine, the eldest, was born in February 1949. I came along precisely one year and one day later, in February 1950. Claudia was born in March of 1954, with Warren arriving eighteen months later in November 1955. The story of my dad is certainly a testament to my mom's courage. Every major life event, i.e., the birth of another child, would soon find Dad crashing headfirst from the platform of mania into an empty pool. My father was diagnosed with manic depression, bipolar 1 with psychosis, as it would be called today. Unfortunately, the best-known treatment for this type of mental illness, lithium, would not be FDA-approved for another fourteen years.

The Peddler

It was fortunate, then, that he was a salesman.

A peddler, he liked to call himself. His first sales job was as a Bible salesman, an interesting career path for a Jew. Well, he converted to Catholicism soon after the birth of his first two children. Even though some years later, he would revert to saying, "Once a Jew, always a Jew."

He found it prophetic when he closed his eyes and put his finger down on this particular job in the classifieds. He was enthused with his newfound religion and, when he went for his interview, was surprised to find that the boss was also a Jew.

"Well, so was Jesus," the boss answered his questioning look.

He approached the pastor of our local Catholic parish, gave him a free Bible and rosary, and received a letter of introduction to the parishioners in return. His sales career was off and running.

Dad was always looking for the right angle. He had to be one step ahead of the pack. Although the Bible sales did not last more than a year, he stayed with that same company for twenty-five years, selling other products with a broader appeal.

For all the years that I can remember, Dad sold silverware in beautiful brown wooden boxes. All the pieces were individually wrapped in tissue paper and placed in their slots of blue felt fabric. The trunk of his car was constantly filled with these heavy boxes. My father's car was the only one in the neighborhood whose tail end was practically dragging on the ground due to the weight in the trunk.

In his own words, Dad said, "There is a gratification that comes with the ability to create a desire in a prospective customer to buy something he had no intention of buying." Yes, he was good. And he thought that highly of himself. The difference between narcissism and being bipolar is that with bipolar disorder, the grandiosity is explicitly seen in episodes of elevated mood, whereas narcissism is an underlying personality style. For me, the jury is still out on whether Dad was bipolar or narcissistic.

He would return from the company's annual banquet with The Salesman of the Year award most years, some silver-plated bowl or wine bucket with his name imprinted. We had a whole collection. These, of course, must have been the manic years.

There was a time when Dad got a parking ticket in Westchester. He had to go to the courthouse to pay the two-dollar fine. In he walked, finely dressed and with a confidence only a hypomanic could exude.

Under his arm was the wooden box containing the Oneida flatware. He paid the bailiff who couldn't help but ask what Dad was carrying. Of course, this was his plan all along, and he immediately went into his sales pitch and convinced the bailiff how happy his wife would be when he brought this box of dinnerware home that night.

It would only be two dollars down and two dollars a week. Without hesitation, he gave Dad back his two-dollar fine as a down payment and thanked him.

This was the 1950s. There was no Walmart or Costco, but there were plenty of supermarkets and factories. Dad thought, why should he go door-to-door selling to one housewife at a time when he could walk into a factory or A&P and sell to dozens at once? He would enter the establishment, offer the manager a free set for letting him solicit there, and gather as many workers as he could to tell them that this was a special offer only for the employees (of whatever company he happened to be in). They didn't even have to put down a deposit. He would leave the flatware sets in the manager's office, and they would only have to pay two dollars a week. The company had collectors who would collect the weekly payments while trying to sell additional products to these customers.

He told me a story about walking into a dress factory in New York City where over a hundred sewing machine operators were having lunch. He stood on top of a high table and asked for their attention. "Ladies," he said, "this is a special offer only for members of Local Eighty-Nine." He had already talked to the foreman and offered her a free set if she would pretend to buy a set of his Oneida flatware in front of her workers. It worked like a charm.

Birth Control

After my father decided to convert to Catholicism, along with his newfound religion and the zealousness that follows the convert, there was the issue of birth control or, rather, the lack thereof, unless you consider the rhythm method a suitable option.

Dad, the proselyte Catholic convert, would, of course, not sin against the rules of his new religion.

In a 1930 pronouncement on birth control, Pope Pius XI declared that contraception was inherently evil and any spouse practicing any act of contraception "violates the law of God and nature" and was "stained by a great and mortal flaw." Condoms, diaphragms, the rhythm method, and even the withdrawal method were forbidden. Only abstinence was permissible to prevent conception. In 1951, the church modified its stance again. Without overturning the prohibition of artificial birth control, Pius XI's successor, Pius XII, deviated from its intent. He approved the rhythm method for couples with "morally valid reasons for avoiding procreation," defining such situations quite broadly. (1)

It is easy in hindsight to gaze in the mirror of the past and watch the unraveling of lives and to calculate that every time another child came into my parents' world, Dad's mania would turn into a deep, dark depression. Six children were born into my family between 1949 and 1966.

My sister Stacey, sixteen years my junior, considers herself culturally Jewish. She didn't go to Catholic school like her older siblings. My parents were very disillusioned with the Catholic Church by that time. She was very close to her Jewish cousins, aunts, and uncles. My mother was an only child, so all our relatives were on my father's Jewish side of the family.

The littlest child took on that cloak of Judaism, though not religiously. She often jokes, "If it were not for Catholicism, I would not be here."

PART 2 – FAMILY SECRETS

MARLENE DUNHAM

Learning the Language

As I grew to adulthood, I would incrementally learn the Family Secrets—too many to learn all at once, too many for a young child to comprehend. Even now, I believe there are un-emerged secrets buried in the cold, hard ground in a Westchester County cemetery where Dad's ashes lie, atop the same grave that holds his eldest daughter's coffin.

At six or seven years old, I understood it was appropriate to be told that Daddy had a stomach problem. It wasn't until years later that I would learn the truth.

I have since discovered this was one of perhaps six or seven major hospitalizations over the years. There was the infamous Bellevue Hospital violent ward, and there were the state institutions with not much of a better reputation—hospitals like Rockland State Hospital in Orangeburg, about thirty miles north of New York City. There were electroshock treatments, straitjackets, isolation, and ribs broken by burly attendants trying to get Dad to cooperate. In the more successful years as a salesman, when his mania worked to his advantage and money was no object, he would find himself in the upper-class mental institutions of New York—hospitals like Gracie Square Hospital on the Upper East Side or Payne Whitney Clinic, where Marilyn Monroe spent time in 1961. Mom always liked to tell us that she saw Eddie Fisher coming out of Payne Whitney when they were there one day. Dad had seen them all.

Another Reality

My father's first hospitalization was most likely in Tucson, Arizona. That would have been after being honorably discharged from the Army in 1945. I know nothing more except that Tucson is where he decided to move his family some thirty years later to get away from the New York creditors looking for him and it was where he died in 1999.

My dad never saved for the bad times. He just spent all he had, and more, during the good times. The older children of the family had a privileged upbringing. There was the summer sleepover camp for two months in the Catskills for three of us. My younger sister was only four years old at the time, but they let her in because her two older sisters were also there. Not just for one summer, but three or four. I can't even imagine what that would cost in today's dollars! There were New York City museums and restaurants, Christmas and Easter shows at Radio City Music Hall, ballet lessons, piano lessons, and more.

The younger children had none of that. They have entirely different perspectives and experiences that shaped their life paths.

His second hospitalization was in 1952 or '53, with two small children at home. The fact that he was at Payne Whitney on the Upper East Side of Manhattan overlooking the East River leads me to believe that he had just come out of a very manic and, therefore, monetarily productive period. Salesmen did not have health benefits, and I've read that the interior of the clinic resembled an upper-middle-class private residence more than a hospital. The poet Robert Lowell wrote of his hospitalization there in several poems.

> After a hearty New England breakfast,
> I weigh two hundred pounds
> this morning. Cock of the walk,
> I strut in my turtle-necked French sailor's jersey
> before the metal shaving mirrors,
> and see the shaky future grow familiar
> in the pinched, indigenous faces of
> these thoroughbred mental cases,
> twice my age and half my weight.
> We are all old-timers,
> each of us holds a locked razor.

> ~ Robert Lowell, *Walking in the Blue*

There are no horror stories of the good hospitals. Dad wrote of his horrific experiences at Bellevue. Still, there are no stories of Payne Whitney or Gracie Square, only that famous people were treated within those hallowed halls. It was almost a source of pride.

Of the 150 short stories my dad wrote and combined in a three-ring binder called *Pieces of My Mind*, one particular story made the most profound impression. It was called Another Reality and told of his six-month stay in the violent ward of Bellevue Hospital following his 'stomach problem.'

The truth of the story was that while at home, watching a TV movie about a man committed to an asylum for twenty years, a psychotic episode ensued. He believed he was actually that TV character and was finding out that his wife had divorced him while he was incarcerated. Not wanting to live the rest of his life with this pain of rejection, Dad went to the kitchen, pulled out a long, sharp knife, and attempted, with both hands, to shove the knife into his heart. He missed his heart and stabbed himself in the stomach instead, saving him from death but landing him in Bellevue's violent ward, sedated for weeks on Thorazine.

I suppose this much was true.

Daddy had a 'stomach problem.'

~~

Dad converted from Judaism to Catholicism around 1955. He took his religious instruction and was baptized by none other than Bishop Fulton J. Sheen at Saint Patrick's Cathedral in New York City. Bishop Sheen had a weekly TV show from 1951–1957 called Life Is Worth Living. He was the first real televangelist. Dad had written to him after watching a few of his shows. He must have been very convincing and in full salesman mode, as the good Bishop invited him down to his office in the city and personally instructed him in the Catholic doctrine. Dad never did anything halfway.

As we all know, there is no one more zealous than a new convert.

So, as he lay in the ambulance that my mother called, hearing the deafening sirens and seeing the blinding red revolving lights reflected off the ceiling, he was praying that he would not die. The reason he wanted to live? Because in his newfound Catholic religion, suicide was a sin. He wanted to live to make amends for the mortal sin he had committed. I wonder, was it a mortal sin if the attempt didn't work? And, in those silent nights, I let my mind drift in that direction. I sometimes wonder if he would have felt the dire need for atonement had he been able to foresee the future when, in a little more than ten years, his eldest daughter would follow through for herself on what was now my father's biggest fear: suicide.

As he told it, when he woke up the next morning in the hospital, he was ecstatic that his prayers had been answered. He was alive, and he would not be going to hell, although all too soon, the realization set in that he was actually in a living hell—the violent ward of Bellevue Hospital. He would spend the next six months there. Diagnosis: Acute paranoia, which only accentuated his abnormal fear of death, a fear that he would die before he repented of the mortal sin he had committed. He knew his suspicions must be correct that the hospital staff was trying to poison his food and his medication.

Thorazine was the drug of choice for the day. It was an antipsychotic. It caused lethargy, emotional numbness, and a significant disconnect from reality. This was not the first time Dad had been hospitalized, so I'm sure he was well acquainted with the effects of Thorazine and did not want to become the zombie it would inevitably turn him into. He had to be on his guard, as he was convinced the staff was trying to kill him with that medication-filled needle. It took three attendants to hold him down. A very large, wrestler-type attendant put Dad in a bear hug while another jabbed him with the needle. This ritual of tackling, wrestling, and bear hugs went on for days until one day, when Dad was especially noncompliant, the bear hug broke three of his ribs and he was sent to a padded cell.

One of the side effects of Thorazine was a parched mouth and swelling of the tongue. Dad was extremely thirsty and dehydrated but still acutely paranoid and convinced his food and drink were poisoned. He knew, even in his delusional state, that if he didn't drink something, he would die.

So, in my demented mind, I did what I thought was a very rational act. I discovered a concave section in the cell's concrete floor and peed into it.

I then crawled like an animal and lapped it up, thus quenching my thirst, realizing that my own urine would be the only liquid that would not poison me.

There was not a lot of healing going on at Bellevue. It had been three or four months; the year had changed to 1960; electroshock therapy was next on the menu. Dad spent that time in fear and despair. He felt he was being imprisoned for a crime rather than hospitalized. Would this be his penance for the crime of attempted suicide? He was utterly dependent on their authority. He wrote of the terror when told by his doctor that he was to undergo electroshock therapy for his depression and paranoia. To Dad, this was synonymous with death in the electric chair.

The following morning, the doctor and three attendants arrayed in white uniforms were waiting for me as I entered the shock therapy room.

I went through the ritual of emptying my bladder, taking two large, red pills with quivering hands. I was then instructed to lay over a pillow placed under the base of my spine. The doctor then applied a sticky paste on the sides of my head, over which were two wires attached to an ugly black box. A fever of anticipation and an agonized unrest hung over me as one of the attendants held my shoulders, another my thighs, and the third inserted a horseshoe shaped object into my mouth and instructed me to take a deep breath, and hold it. My eyes were constantly glued to the black, sinister-looking box awaiting apprehensively the pull of the handle that would send countless volts crashing through my brain.

After what seemed a fraction of a second, I opened my eyes to find the doctor staring at me. Thinking the treatment had not begun, I asked when he would start.

He said, 'My boy, we finished about an hour ago.'

You have no idea how relieved I was to know I was alive.

I must say, I was also relieved to read my dad's account of his electroshock therapy because my research brought to life scenarios more like what we read in the pages of *One Flew Over The Cuckoo's Nest*. According to the Mayo Clinic, shock therapy in the 1950s was given by "sending a very strong electric current from temple to temple of the patient." Since no anesthetics were used, broken bones were a common occurrence for some from the powerful seizures.

Dad had over a hundred electroshock treatments during those years of hospitalizations.

33

Lithium

Lithium is a natural salt. Lithium-ion = Li+. Some say it has been used since Roman times in the form of spring water. However, it was not approved for use as a drug in the U.S. until 1970 because the pharmaceutical industry did not want to invest in a drug that could not be patented.

There was no money to be made, and it was cheap.

It was about 1964 when we moved out of Hudson Gardens, only to go about a block away. My father wanted more space for some reason, probably because he was manic and had lots of money. We rented two apartments right next to each other, and we were permitted to knock down the connecting wall. The kids' side had two bedrooms, a bathroom, and a kitchen that we never used. My bedroom window was at ground level, so my sister and I had friends climb through the window without our parents ever knowing until one day when they were watching from the patio on the other end of the apartment.

A year later, my older sister was in a hospital in Manhattan; my father was in Bellevue again; my brother was in Willowbrook. We couldn't afford two apartments anymore. I can only assume that my well-to-do grandparents paid our bills during Dad's absence. I never really thought about where the money came from. At fourteen, there were more important things to think about. I was, however, the only one old enough to support my mother emotionally and physically. So, we packed up the apartments, and back to Hudson Gardens we went.

34

Claudia was ten, and my brother Bruce was three. The littlest, Stacey, would not be born for another two years, and in three years, by 1967, my older sister would be dead.

~~

In the 1960s, a lithium underground developed in the United States as physicians began prescribing the drug without Food and Drug Administration approval. (1) Since lithium is a natural element, it could not be patented—and thus, the drug companies had little interest in pursuing it as a treatment. There was no profit to be made. Nevertheless, Dr. Ronald Fieve and several other researchers convinced the FDA to approve lithium as a treatment for manic depression in 1970. (2)

My research uncovered the fact that Bellevue Hospital was doing clinical trials as early as 1963. This was when Dr. Samuel Gershon became the head of the Neuropsychopharmacology Unit at New York University. Ronald Fieve, M.D., and colleagues at the New York State Psychiatric Hospital conducted the first systematic study on the effectiveness of lithium. They set up the first lithium clinic in North America at Columbia University in 1966. (3)

They evaluated nineteen patients who were unsuccessfully treated with phenothiazines or electro-convulsive therapy. Serendipity? Synchronicity? Dad was in the right place at the right time, whether at Bellevue, Rockland State, or Columbia Presbyterian, where trials were going on. All I know is that Dad was starting lithium trials by my sixteenth birthday in 1966. Like any new drug, there was trial and error. My sister committed suicide in 1967, which sent him into another tailspin, and it took another year or two for him to become stabilized. I never did the math until I was in my forties. That is when I realized I had lived with an unmedicated manic depressive father for the first sixteen or seventeen years of my life. I would be out of the house for good in little more than two years. So that's all I ever knew. Insanity.

Dr. Fieve states, "We really don't know how lithium works." But before lithium, all we had was lobotomy, electroconvulsive therapy, and Thorazine. One of his patients said, "Mania was my first love, and it's very, very hard to give up." It's a hard thing to consistently stay on lithium. When you're in a manic state, you don't want to come out of it, and there is little fear of falling. You are invincible.

My dad always told me that it was a mixed blessing to be manic-depressive. In his manic state, there was a "total absence of fear, rocketed into an ecstatic high, suddenly transformed from a fearful, vulnerable, puny excuse for a man ... to a superman." It gave him the confidence that he needed to become such a successful salesman. When he was manic, he was invincible.

While in the depths of depression, he equated it to being in an emotional straitjacket (albeit sometimes that was literal), incapable of doing even the simplest tasks. He lived those days in hopelessness and fear. But my dad always said he could endure the suffering because that was the price he had to pay to experience the heights of euphoria. In his own words: "I grieve over the loss of my mania."

PART 3 - INSTITUTIONS

Not Forgotten

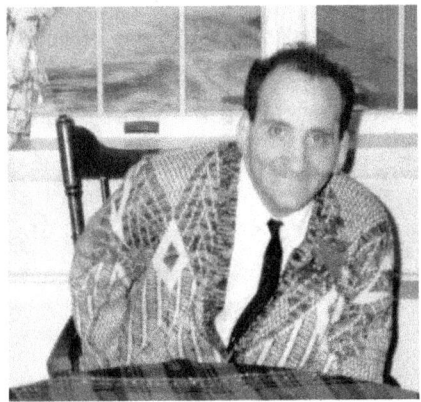

His name is Warren, and he is what they used to call 'profoundly retarded,' which I know is no longer politically correct. He is an individual with a severe intellectual disability, and he is my brother.

Warren was born in 1955 and was the first boy after three girls.

He is five years my junior, and to be perfectly honest, before this writing project, I did not think of him very often. I had not seen Warren in over fifty years.

I began corresponding, a term I use loosely, as Warren does not write. He does not speak. His IQ hovers below 20, and he does not know who I am, an excuse I saw my parents embrace most of their lives to alleviate the guilt of no contact, of giving up their parenthood, when it came to their fourth child and firstborn son.

To be fair to my parents, it's what you did in the 1950s. Your pediatrician suggested it, and all the specialists recommended it. Many families faced these same choices. For some, it was a deep, dark family secret, not even knowing that their siblings, or relative even existed. For others, there would be weekly visits to whichever institution. I know it wasn't easy for any of them.

As of this writing, I plan to visit my brother in his group home near Plattsburgh, New York, along with my sister, Stacey, who has never met her brother. He is sixty-eight years old. She is fifty-seven. When she was born, Warren had already been institutionalized for ten years. Family visits had pretty much ended by then. She can't even remember when she first discovered she had another brother. It may have been around the same time she found out she had another sister—not until her early teens!

Warren was approximately two years old when it became increasingly evident that something was wrong. He would spend hours sitting on the floor, with his head against the wall, rocking back and forth, back and forth. His hair had worn a little bald patch in the spot where it met the plaster. Words were not spoken. Words were echoed, much like a parrot mimicking immediately after hearing them. No words came out of their own accord. No babbling two-year-old banter, the type we parents sometimes complain about. I'm sure there was no complaining by my parents. Only worry. Enough worry to make appointment after appointment with specialist after specialist. Diagnosis: Severe Mental Retardation. Age three.

My father was manic-depressive in the days before lithium. I have often thought, "What would I have done?"

With three children of my own (all born within twenty-seven months of each other), I've often pondered that question. There are those who say that the parents were ashamed. Others say they just threw their children away and forgot about them. I don't pretend to know the answer.

The Benches was where all the mothers of the building would meet with their toddlers and their strollers to socialize and gossip. It was a long strip of a park adjacent to Henry Hudson Parkway with benches extending a city block. I remember playing there as a child with dozens of other kids from the building. I have very few memories of my childhood, but The Benches I always remember as a safe place. I have had recurring dreams in my adult life of various scenarios where someone is chasing me, trying to kill me, etc. I always knew that if I could just get back to The Benches and lay down on the concrete—I would always wake up in my bed. I would be safe.

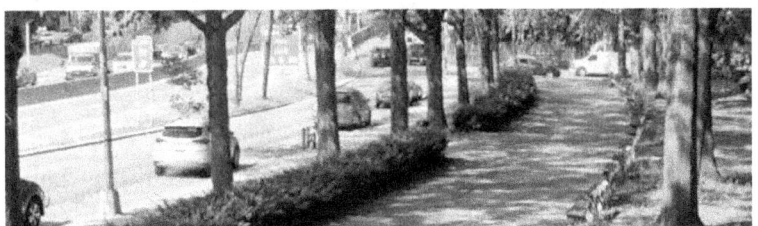

The Benches

Mom was embarrassed to have the other moms at The Benches see her son, who was not quite normal, so instead of her usual routine with the older children, of going to The Benches with the other mothers, she would take Warren in the stroller and walk for hours, she told me, so her baby would not be seen, and apparently, she would not be embarrassed. It was the 1950s, but it is still hard for me to fathom.

The doctors, the specialists, and even the Catholic priests would all weigh in. It was decided that the best thing for all would be to place Warren in a home for the mentally ill.

At least Dad was going through a manic stage at the time. He was a salesman working on full commission. These were years when the family had lots of money!

The decision was made that Warren, not yet four years old, would be sent to one of the best and, I'm sure, most expensive private institutions in the Greater New York area. The place was called Ferncliff Manor on Saw Mill River Parkway in Yonkers; I remember driving north, up that tree-lined parkway along the river every Sunday afternoon to visit Warren. I was eight.

We would go to the Carvel ice cream stand down the road. Sad but true, this is the only concrete memory I have of my brother. Carvel on Sundays.

Unfortunately, what goes up must come down. The mania of my father, along with his record-breaking sales performance, came crashing down. He was hospitalized, and the income dried up.

The private institution had to give way to a state mental hospital.

Those may be the three most dreaded words in the English language.

Warren was transferred to Willowbrook State Hospital on Staten Island. It was actually called a school, and it was the largest institution for the developmentally disabled in the world at the time (and that was not a good thing).

Willowbrook

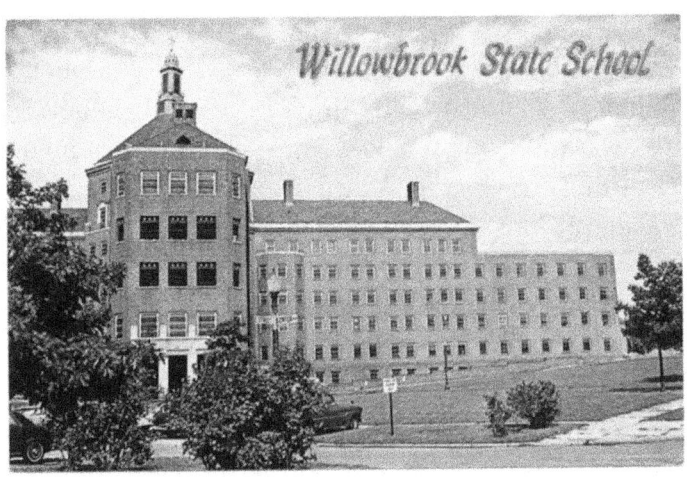

Willowbrook State School (New York Public Library)

Initially built in 1942, it first opened as a United States Army Hospital called Halloran General Hospital. It resembled a college campus, surrounded by brick buildings and grassy areas spread out on a tract of about 375 acres on Staten Island. In October 1947, the New York State Department of Mental Hygiene took it over and opened it as The Willowbrook State School, New York City's institution for people with developmental disabilities. It was built to hold 4,000, but by 1965, there were over 6,200 residents. (1)

My brother spent about fifteen years of his life at Willowbrook, the place that Robert F. Kennedy called "a snake pit" in 1965. When Kennedy visited the site, he was horrified by what he saw and stated that "individuals in the overcrowded facility were living in filth and dirt, their clothing in rags, in rooms less comfortable and cheerful than the cages in which we put animals in a zoo." (2)

Overcrowding and understaffing are what compiled the problems of Willowbrook. I don't necessarily believe that there was intentional abuse and neglect, although, in institutions such as these, and human nature being what it is, such things do happen. If intentional neglect were to have a target, I would hurl it at the New York State Department of Mental Hygiene.

A combination of budget cuts by Governor Nelson Rockefeller and more demand for placements coupled with indifference led to most of Willowbrook's problems. Some quote a ratio of seventy patients to two or three caregivers. I wonder how those caregivers could keep clothes on the backs of children with mental disabilities as severe as most residents, who would disrobe as fast as staff could dress them? How could they keep the feces and urine cleaned up when there were seventy other children to look after?

Willowbrook was also the place that began the career of a relatively unknown investigative reporter for WABC TV in New York in 1972 named Geraldo Rivera. He broke the story of the abuse and filth of this institution and started the ball rolling on what has been called the "single largest venture in deinstitutionalization." (3)

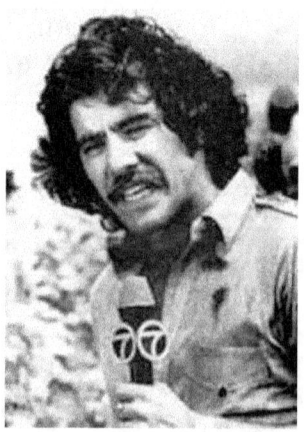

Geraldo Rivera Reporting from Willowbrook, 1972

Geraldo had been friends with a doctor who worked at Willowbrook, Dr. Michael Wilkins. Dr. Wilkins came to New York in 1967 to complete his medical residency as a pediatric intern and was recruited to Willowbrook by a friend also working there at the time. In an interview with Dr. Wilkins in 2007, he tells how he began organizing parents and letting them know what was really going on behind closed doors. (4) Since parents and friends were not allowed in the buildings, they held Sunday barbeques outside. There, they would advocate for improvement in the conditions. These meetings eventually led to a conference for the parents. The keynote speaker, an expert on mental retardation, described conditions at Willowbrook as "primitive" and "outdated." (4)

In the interview, Wilkins said,

The first thing that assaults you when you walk in the building is the smell, and that sets the tone for the whole experience. The smell is the smell of decay and a mixture of sweat and feces and lack of being cleansed, it permeated the building. (4)

The clients spent their days in the dayroom. Most were heavily medicated to keep their energy levels down.

It wasn't a school at all. Their life is just hours and hours of endless nothing to do.

For the incontinent, the attendants would get six to eight clients together in the shower room and hose them to keep them clean and clean up after them between showers. The severely retarded would be on the floor in straitjackets so as not to scratch themselves or assault other patients. Some would rock on the floor, while others sat motionless.

Parents did not see this Willowbrook. The families that did come to visit were not allowed into the dayrooms or the sleeping quarters, where up to seventy beds were lined up in the back rooms with hardly any space between them. The residents had no personal possessions.

The family would come to the front door, and their child would be brought to them. They would be dressed up and cleaned up.

Dr. Wilkins, along with his friend Dr. Bronston, began advocating for change. Governor Nelson Rockefeller had just instituted large budget cuts that eliminated staff at Willowbrook, which was already insufficient. They held Sunday meetings outside on the grounds with the parents who were interested. They even let them into the back rooms to see for themselves.

After only seventeen months working at Willowbrook, Dr. Wilkins was fired for his efforts to organize parents. Fortunately, when he was fired, they had never asked for his keys. This is when he contacted his friend Geraldo and let him and his camera crew in to document the place for posterity and to change history.

> Never doubt that a small group of thoughtful, committed citizens can change the world. Indeed, it is the only thing that ever has.
>
> ~ Margaret Mead

Geraldo won a Peabody Award for this investigation, which garnered national attention and eventually led to the 1972 Consent Decree (6) and the closing of Willowbrook State School forever.

Here is a copy of the letter that my mother wrote to Geraldo in January of 1972, just a week after his undercover reporting:

January 14, 1972

Dear Mr. Rivera,

    I salute you and bless you for your coverage, this past week, of the desparate situation at Willowbrook and the other State "Schools." Your dedication and humanity certainly was instrumental in waking up the hearts of our fellow New Yorkers.

    I am a free-lance writer who has tried, (in vain) to bring this story to any small segment of the public. More than that, infinitely so - I am the mother of Warren, a retarded child who lives, or rather exists at Willowbrook.

    Warren is our fourth child of six and is profoundly retarded. He has been at Willowbrook for a little more tha n a year. Before that, for twelve years, my husba nd and I provided for Warren's care at Ferncliff Manor, Yonkers, N.Y., one of the few wonderful private institutions with a director and staff profoundly dedicated to the welfare of the retarded.

    Unfortunate illnesses and conseque nt fina ncial reve rses in so la rge a family, brought us, against our will, to the "ultimate solution" - the Sta te .

    We were all to cognizant of the late Sena tor Kennedy's investigation of Willowbrook in the early 1960's. (How many remember it now, though, Geraldo?)

    Presently, ou r son is a patient at Bellevue Hospital, transferred there, temporarily from Willowbrook, on December 15, suffering from cuts, bleeding and abrasions of the bla dder. Imagine our shock when the doctor told us that in addition an insect had been found in his bladder. We, personally attribute this situation to the lack of care at Willowbrook. Of course, no one will admit that, neither Ward D of the Infirmary in Building #2 or Warren's regular "home " at Building # 8.

    In any event, we are without recourse and at the mercy of existing circumstances. Along with so many, we are helpless and heart-broken.

Yours most sincerely,

Joan Halper
(Mrs. Burton Howard Halper)

Willowbrook lost a class-action suit against the State of New York. The court case took three years. It represented 5,400 residents of Willowbrook and was filed in federal court. In 1975, The Willowbrook Consent Decree was signed that committed New York State to improve community placement for the now designated Willowbrook Class. (5)

The Willowbrook Class represented any person in residence as of March 17, 1972, as was my brother. The judgment was twenty-nine pages long, and it pledged that New York State would reduce the population of Willowbrook from 5,400 to no more than 250 by 1987.

On February 25, 1987, the federal court approved the Willowbrook 1987 Stipulation, setting forth guidelines for providing community placements for class members. (5)

The Willowbrook School was closed that year.

Although the Consent Decree of 1972 did not require complete closure of the facility, it established that residents of Willowbrook had a constitutional right to be protected from harm and required NY state to take immediate steps to improve the lives of those who lived there and to "ready each resident ... for life in the community at large" and called for the placement of Willowbrook residents in the "least restrictive and most normal living conditions possible." These included ensuring residents were provided with basic necessities like clothing, and opportunities to leave their beds, interact with the community, and be provided with therapy and vocational services. (6)

Thanks to people like Dr. Wilkins, Dr. Bronston, and Geraldo Rivera, the exposure of the problems at Willowbrook and its subsequent closure has directly led to legislation such as the 1975 Developmental Disabilities Assistance and Bill of Rights Act, the Education for All Handicapped Children Act and the Civil Rights of Institutionalized Persons Act of 1980 and which led to the 1990 passage of the Americans with Disabilities Act (ADA). The closure of Willowbrook not only returned the disabled to the community where they belonged, but it also was the catalyst in the deinstitutionalization process throughout New York state and the United States.

Since my brother was a resident of Willowbrook in 1972, my parents would have been among the parents of the 5,400 people living there, which this court case represented. Interestingly, when I asked my mother about the case, she said she knew nothing of the lawsuit. I find that amazing. And a bit disturbing.

She went on to say that she and my father were also on a Parents Committee and never actually saw the neglect and abuse that was talked about. Obviously, this was not the same parents committee organized by Dr. Wilkins.

I don't remember my mother going to Willowbrook more than once or twice. I myself went once and never went back. It was a creepy place. I have not seen my brother in over fifty years. Her recollection never quite aligned with the actual truth in the letter she wrote to Geraldo. I have attributed this to the mother I remember, who always liked to avoid reality and not remember things as they were, but as she would have liked them to be.

In a portion of that 1972 letter from my mother to Geraldo Rivera, she wrote:

Presently, our son is a patient at Bellevue Hospital, transferred there temporarily from Willowbrook on December 15, suffering cuts, bleeding, and abrasions of the bladder. Imagine our shock when the doctor told us that, in addition, an insect had been found in his bladder.

There may still, to this day, be much secrecy about what went on at Willowbrook State School up until 1987. Still, great strides have been made in the years since in treating and non-institutionalizing the mentally handicapped in the United States. I am lucky to know where my brother is today. Some never discovered what happened to their loved ones. It seems that many had been transferred out of Willowbrook, without a trace. Thousands of children died at Willowbrook, and their families don't know where their loved ones are buried. I have read accounts of families that do not know if their relative is dead or alive. I am so thankful that I know where my brother is today and I know that he is being well cared for.

After Willowbrook

Since 1985, at the age of thirty, my brother has been living in a group home in upstate New York. The Consumer Advisory Board (CAB) monitors his well-being, which provides necessary and appropriate representation and advocacy services on an individual basis for all Willowbrook Class members as long as any class member lives.

There are several ways Willowbrook Class members can be represented. A Class member can advocate for themselves or have a co-representative such as a family member, advocate, or the Consumer Advisory Board (CAB). They can also choose full representation from a family member, Advocate, or the CAB. Representation is first and foremost for the class member.

If the family is not meeting the standard of active representation, for whatever reason, and the Class member cannot self-advocate, then the member should be referred to CAB. My parents would have received a letter similar to the one below.

Dear [Correspondent]:

I am writing to advise you of the availability of the Consumer Advisory Board (CAB), which advocates for Willowbrook class members. With the signing of the Willowbrook Consent Judgment, the CAB was designated to act "in loco parentis" (in place of the parent) for Willowbrook class members who have no involved family. In addition, the CAB is available to provide co-representation for family members who are unable to provide "active representation," as required by the Willowbrook Permanent Injunction, i.e., participation with the program team in planning and evaluating the individual development plan and/or visits at least annually.

If you believe that assistance from the CAB would be a benefit for your (state relationship), please return the enclosed form, which details your options for representation, co-representation, or no participation by the CAB. Co-representation would provide the CAB with the power to advocate on behalf of (class member name), by attending case conferences and ensuring that his/her rights are not violated. You, however, retain the responsibility for signing all necessary documents and consent forms. If you select full representation by the CAB, local staff will attend case conferences and advocate for (class member name), and also sign documents on behalf of your (state relationship). You would in no way be giving up any of your rights as family, and may revoke your choice at any time.

If you have any questions or concerns, please contact me at (phone number). Your prompt response would be most beneficial to (class member name).

Thank you for your cooperation in ensuring active representation for (class member name).

My parents either signed the forms to have their son represented by the Board, or they did not reply at all. Either way, fortunately, Warren has been well-taken care of for the past thirty-eight years of his life. He has his own advocate on the CAB who makes sure that all the stipulations of the Willowbrook Decree are being followed when it comes to someone from the Willowbrook Class, as is my brother. But I often wonder, what about the trauma of the past? What does he remember? What does he comprehend of the horrors of growing up in an institution such as Willowbrook? I am in contact with his advocate as well as his local caseworker.

They say he seems happy but does tend to withdraw and isolate himself. He doesn't trust people very much. I suppose I can't blame him. I only pray that when I go for my first visit in fifty years, he will have a sense of who I am, a recognition that we belong together somehow, like pieces of the puzzle that was once our family.

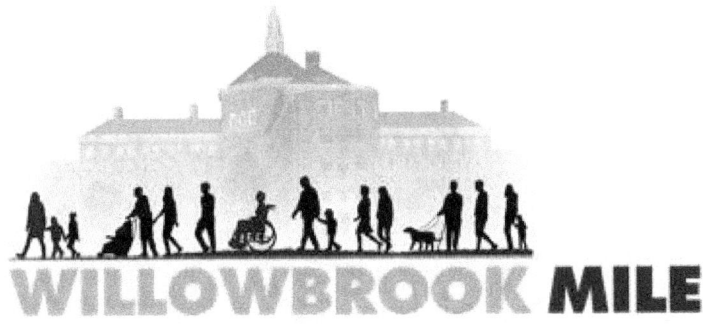

The Path Forward is a film released in 2022 by the New York State Developmental Disabilities Planning Council, commemorating fifty years since Geraldo Rivera's exposure of Willowbrook State School in 1972. It highlights the importance of lessons learned, the positive changes that have resulted in the past fifty years, and to make sure that it never happens again.

The College of Staten Island (CUNY) is now located on the site of Willowbrook. Instead of hiding the atrocities that happened on this land, to their credit, motivated by the conviction that it should never be forgotten and that nothing like this should ever happen again, they have embraced it, educated the community, and built a

Memorial Walking Trail called the Willowbrook Mile, consisting of twelve stations that mark the history of the site, with benches and landscaping. It opened officially on September 17, 2022, the thirty-fifth anniversary of the closing of Willowbrook. This unique project aims to preserve the site's history and create a visionary presence commemorating the continuing struggle for social justice for all people of all abilities.

Not Forgotten—Part 2

The semi-annual reports from The Dept of Disability Service Office (DDSO) all start the same.

Warren is a handsome gentleman with dark hair, eyes, and a smile that can light up a room.

Warren's smile is contagious. Warren can say a few words, but this is only on a rare occasion. Although Warren is nonverbal, he is able to express his emotions, wants, needs, and desires in a nonverbal way through actions, body language, gestures, and some sign language.

In another paragraph, it says that Warren is "electively mute."

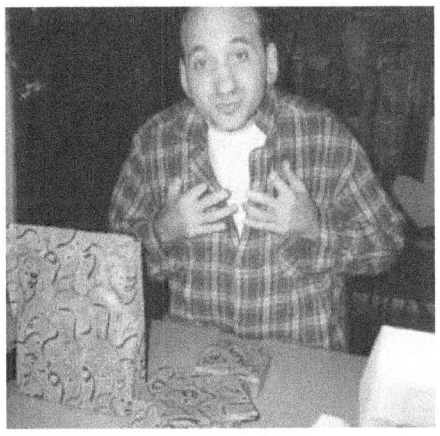

Warren is saying, "Please, may I open my gifts?"

Not mentioned here is that Warren is missing the tops of at least six fingers, and, sometime in the past, his nose had been broken. Warren also has no teeth. I read an account of a Willowbrook parent stating that the

Willowbrook dentist was notorious for pulling teeth. Her child had no teeth because she would bite herself until she bled. Whether this is connected with Warren's missing fingers or missing teeth or is a result of abuse or self-mutilation remains a mystery. Geraldo even reported that he does not remember seeing toothbrushes in the wards. Not surprisingly, records from Willowbrook don't seem to exist. We'll never know.

I'm told he loves music. That must be a family trait—one of the good things we share. Music has meant so much to me my whole life, even though I don't play an instrument. Our brother Bruce has been a drummer for the past forty or so years. My parents were lovers of music, too. Warren loves classic rock—a man after my own heart. Music therapy is essential in the lives of the mentally disabled, probably because music is nonverbal. It transcends language. Hans Christian Anderson once said, "Where words fail, music speaks." My brother is nonverbal, and I like to think that the music he listens to speaks to him in some way. I know that it calms us down, not just as therapy but for all of us music lovers, it calms anxieties and relaxes us when we are overstimulated.

> Music has healing power. It has the ability to
> take people out of themselves for a few hours.
>
> ~ Elton John

I'm told he can spend hours sitting in a rocking chair on the back porch of his home in Plattsburgh listening to his CDs. His caseworker has told me the porch is Warren's Man Cave and no one usually goes there except him. He has his favorite chair and weighted blanket and will rock and listen to his music. His favorite group is the Beatles and, in particular, John Lennon. An interesting fact I did not know until I was researching for this book:

According to Wikipedia: "After John Lennon watched (Geraldo) Rivera's report on the patients at Willowbrook, he and Rivera formed a benefit concert called *One to One.*"

Serendipity, do you think?

In 2002, the semi-annual report I received from DDSO said:

Warren has a history of stealing food. Warren is cautious of new people and often displays maladaptive behaviors to see what he can get away with. Since he is nonverbal, he doesn't have the ability to tell anyone if an abusive situation has occurred. Warren can become physically aggressive towards others if they are between him and an object he is focused on.

Warren has the potential for self-abusive behaviors, such as eating and drinking nonedible items.

Staff should be aware that he often grabs hot liquids or items cooking on the stove and may try to consume them. He should remain within eyesight at all times while in the kitchen.

OCD is another diagnosis of Warren's. I find this one interesting in that family members around me seem to have a lot of OCD tendencies.

Warren has some OCD behaviors that keep him very active. He likes everything to be in its correct place, such as furniture being arranged in a particular way, the phone hanging up in a certain way, and the curtains hanging 'just so.' He keeps things in order. He can be quite helpful in clearing things away, such as mats after PT, arranging and clearing the living room after various activities. In the past, there has been some concern that his arranging and organizing sometimes intruded on activities that were in progress!

This brought a smile to my face!

From the 2006 Annual Report, it shows dramatic improvement.

Social isolation and withdrawal continue to be a major concern in his overall adjustment. He continues to spend a considerable amount of time apart from the main group, typically engaged in some rocking-type behavior. However, his current status still shows significant progress over the patterns of adjustment Warren displayed during the earlier years of placement. His overall behavior adjustment had improved dramatically over the years and certainly, since his placement in Clinton County began. [1986]

Warren tends to choose people he will trust when going out into the community. He will show greater participation when with them. He greets others by shaking their hand; however, he does not initiate this action. Warren often makes his acquaintance with others by gently touching their ears.

A recent note from his caregiver stated,

He is doing well. Has calmed down a lot over the years and seems to be happy. Smiles and laughs often.

I guess that's all you can ask for. He grew up in Willowbrook.

Warren has a personal savings account that cannot accumulate over $2,000. When the account gets up there, they go shopping to spend it down. His basic needs are taken care of, so he can shop for things he especially likes. His caregiver said Warren has the most expensive taste of any man she's ever met. They will go to J.C. Penney's, and he will go directly to the silk shirts or the most expensive items they sell.

Warren is a very interesting and complex person who is very in tune with his environment. At times, his way of exploring the environment can run contrary to accepted procedures and safety factors.

I love how they call Warren a very "interesting and complex" person. It shows the respect that he garners as a person, not simply as someone or something to be taken care of. Not forgotten.

And now I have told the story of my brother—the person—Warren. For those of you reading my story, consider that your ears have been gently touched by my brother.

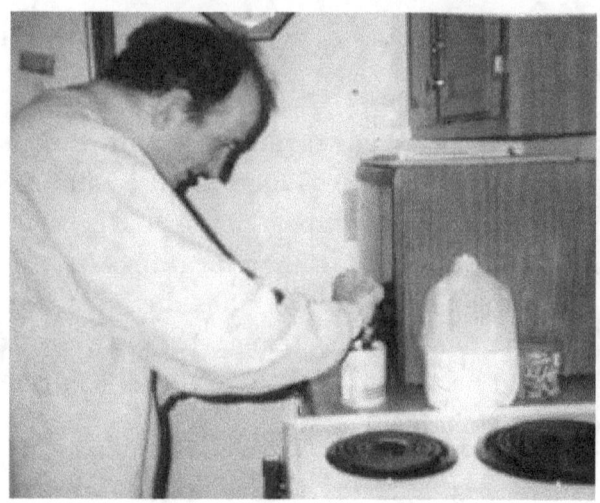

"Warren is capable of making himself a cup of instant coffee and using the microwave."

PART 4 – DIFFERENT PERSPECTIVES

MARLENE DUNHAM

Lorraine

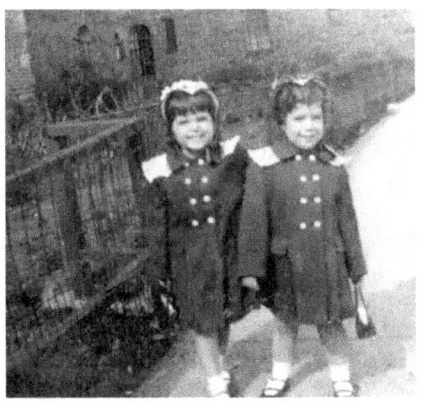

1954 L-R Lorraine and-Me

It was so long ago. Fifty years.

In many ways, it seems like a story that I read or perhaps a movie that stayed with me and haunted me, but the memory is still so real. It's different for everyone: the loss of a loved one, the loss of a sibling. It doesn't matter if this sibling was a small child or an adult or if the death was caused by a freak accident or a fatal disease. It is hard, no matter what the circumstances.

Lorraine and I were one year and one day apart. She was born on February 22, 1949. I came along on February 23, 1950, at 2:10am, so just barely what they call Irish Twins, siblings born within twelve months of each other. I was always a little bigger and taller, so we looked like twins. It didn't hurt that our parents always dressed us in matching outfits. There were matching black velvet dresses at Christmas time and pink flowered dresses at

Easter. My poor sister, four years younger, would get two of every hand-me-down.

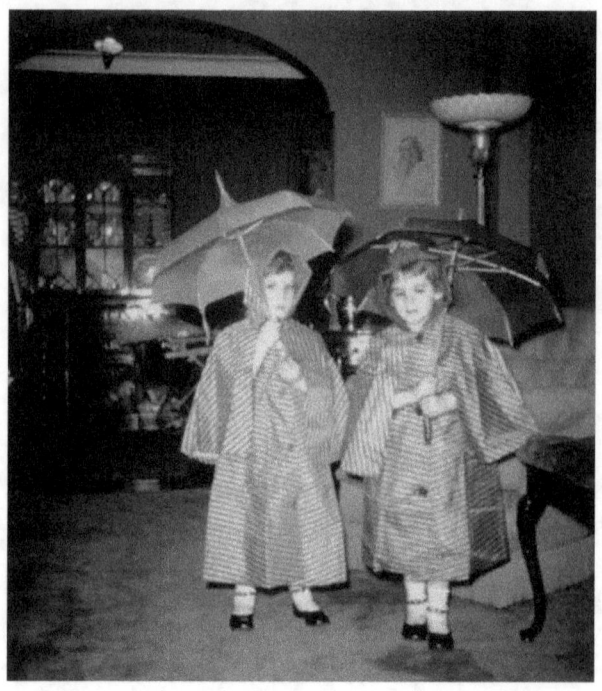

I get a kick out of looking at these early pictures, as I not only have twin daughters myself but twin granddaughters as well.

I suppose we were close as children. I don't really remember. I don't remember a lot of things about my childhood. If a coping mechanism from childhood trauma is protecting me or just old age memory loss, I don't know. There certainly was trauma.

We grew apart as we grew older and into pre-teen and teenage years. I always thought she was a bit square, in the vernacular of the '60s.

My sister Lorraine died when she was eighteen years old.

I was seventeen.

It started to become apparent that there was a problem when she was about fourteen or fifteen. Lorraine became distant, confused, and disoriented. She dropped out of high school because she couldn't concentrate. Being one year younger and a teenager at the time, I thought she was a bit different, so I would go my own way, do my own thing, and not have much to do with my slightly older sister. It's so unfortunate that the young can be so uncompassionate. I have always felt guilty for my apathy.

SUMMER - 1965

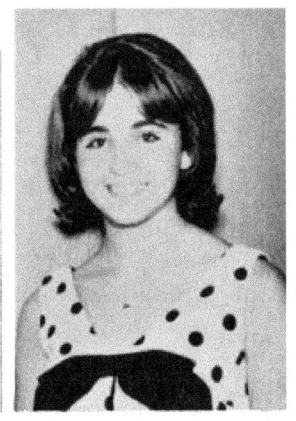

Miss Halper Enters Teenager Contest

Lorraine Halper, 16, daughter of Mr. and Mrs. Burton Halper of 2728 Henry Hudson Parkway, was a semi-finalist in the Miss American Teenager contest held at Palisade Park last week.

Miss Halper is a junior at Walton High School and plans to enter junior college with a view toward a Peace Corps career. This is the first contest she has entered. The competition was based on personality and looks.

Lorraine was beautiful. In 1965, at age fifteen, she entered the Miss Teenage America Pageant that took place each year at Palisades Park in Fort Lee, New Jersey. We could practically see the park from our bedroom window on the other side of the Hudson River, just above the cliffs—the Palisades. There was no talent competition. The competition was based on personality and looks. She advanced to the semi-finals. The newspaper clipping says that she had a view toward a Peace Corps career. I didn't know that.

The following year, she entered the Miss Riverdale Contest in our town. I can't remember the outcome, but I

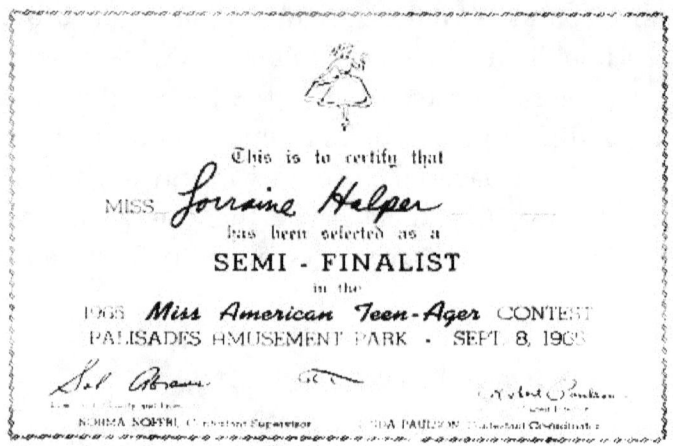

do remember her receiving several prizes, including a set of professional photos from a local photographer.

Years later, those photos hanging in our parents' home would bring my youngest sister to ask, "Who is that girl?" when she was about seven years old. Apparently, no one had yet told her about Lorraine.

After a year of boarding school, where my parents thought the Sisters of Mercy could help, she came home to the first of a half dozen or so stays at different New York mental hospitals. Her diagnosis: schizophrenia.

Some of these hospital stays would coincide with those of Dad—different hospitals, different diagnoses.

Schizophrenia occurs in all cultures and societies. While the exact cause is unknown, research suggests that there is a combination of genetic, psychological, and environmental factors.

Symptoms of schizophrenia develop slowly over time. The average age of onset tends to be in the late teens to the early thirties, but signs might even be seen in early teen years. It can be challenging to diagnose schizophrenia in teens because the first signs can look like typical adolescent behavior, like a change of friends, a drop in grades, sleep problems, and irritability. Other factors include isolating oneself and withdrawing from others, an increase in unusual thoughts and suspicions, and a family history of psychosis.

According to the National Alliance on Mental Illness (NAMI) (1), Schizophrenia isn't caused by just one genetic variation, but by a complex interplay of genetics and environmental influences. Heredity does play a strong role. Your likelihood of developing schizophrenia is more than six times higher if you have a close relative with the disorder, such as a parent or sibling. This fact has always led me to ask what the connection would be between bipolar 1 and schizophrenia.

On a weekend pass, I vividly remember her sitting in our living room telling my parents she had something very important to say. We all listened to her intently as she announced that she was pregnant. Shock came over all of us. We sat with our mouths open, speechless, as she continued to tell us her story. She told us that she was the Virgin Mary and this baby would be the baby Jesus. Well, needless to say, our mouths remained open, but now for very different reasons.

It was not long after that when she went through her catatonic state, unaware of her surroundings and unresponsive. A common theme in schizophrenia is religious psychosis, which is a complicated issue in itself.

Persons with severe and persistent mental illness and approximately 25–39% of patients with schizophrenia and 15–22% of those with mania/bipolar have religious delusions.

Religious delusions are associated with a more severe course of illness and poorer outcomes. Research has shown that patients with religious delusions had more severe psychotic symptoms, a longer history of illness, and poorer functioning prior to the onset of a psychotic episode. (2)

There are certainly distinctions between psychosis and spiritual experience.

Thomas Szasz, a psychiatrist whose 1961 book *The Myth of Mental Illness* questioned the legitimacy of his field and provided the intellectual grounding for generations of critics, patient advocates, and antipsychiatry activists, making enemies of many fellow doctors, (3). He is known for the quote:

If you talk to God, you are praying; If God talks to you, you have schizophrenia. (3)

Hmm ... A discussion for another time.

Szasz did not deny that humans have difficulties, but he preferred to see them not as mental illnesses or as diseases but as problems in living.

All I know is that too many members of my family had problems in living.

Lorraine's next hospital stay was much more extended. I can remember on a few occasions she would call me and tell me that she was suicidal. We talked for hours, and she usually felt much better when we were done. Obviously, I also felt better for having helped. I had somehow found a little more compassion for my sister. The last of these calls was a week before her death. I was supposed to visit her that weekend, however, I chose to hang out with friends rather than visit my sister in the mental hospital.

I am at peace with the reality that it was not my fault. My visit would not have quieted the demons in her mind. She was not reaching out for help. She was looking for finality.

I came home from school to meet the local church pastor at the elevator to our apartment.

My first thought was that something was wrong with Lorraine; otherwise, why would Father Boyle be standing at the elevator? It was a long and silent ride to the eighth floor. When I walked into the house, my mother hugged me and continued crying, which she had obviously been doing for a while.

My sister had died. Lorraine ran away from the mental hospital on Staten Island, hopped on a subway to Greenwich Village, ran into a building, and jumped.

It was a long time ago. Fifty years. In those fifty years, I have read many books on schizophrenia. To the best of my mental capability, I have learned what it must have been like for her, and I have also let go of the guilt I felt for not visiting her that day in the hospital.

It was not until over forty years later, however, that I learned what happened that day in Greenwich Village. And I found it out from the unlikeliest of sources: my youngest sister, who was only a year old when Lorraine died.

Stacey and Claudia

Stacey grew up among pictures of this very pretty girl scattered around on the walls of our apartment. The photos were of when she had won the Miss Riverdale Contest.

Stacey told me,

When I was about six or seven years old, I finally asked my parents , 'Who is this girl in all these black and white photographs around the house?' The answer was simple: 'Oh, she was your sister,' to which I then asked, 'Oh, then where is she?' I imagine my parents were waiting for this to be asked before freely offering this information on their own. 'Oh, she got sick and died,' was the reply. I took in this information, put two and two together, and thought to myself, Perhaps I too will get sick and suddenly die. I had no memory of this phantom sister, as I was only eighteen months old when she died. I imagine I either knew better or was afraid to ask more questions. The subject never arose again. I soon developed quite an anxiety disorder with this new and incomplete information. My first panic attack was at about age eleven. Frequent anxiety attacks continued beyond my college years.

It wasn't for about another seven years that I would find out the rest of the story. The family had moved to Tucson, Arizona, in 1974. The two older girls were already living on their own, but Claudia moved out to Tucson a few years later. She had an apartment near my high school, and I was visiting one day after school. A day I will never forget. The subject of Lorraine came up, and I asked the question I had wanted to ask for years. 'How did Lorraine die?'

'What?' she angrily replied—'no one ever told you?' She couldn't believe it.

I told her that no one ever discussed it again after I asked about the black and white photos in the New York apartment when I was seven.

She told me that Lorraine was mentally ill. She was in and out of institutions and one day ran away from the hospital into New York City and jumped from a building. I don't remember if she mentioned schizophrenia, but now I had something else to worry about. Perhaps I, too, will become mentally ill.

Stacey had many issues regarding this family secret. (As a parent, I can somehow understand thinking you are shielding your child from the evil of the world, but it never works out that way.)

She also does not remember ever being told about her brother Warren. And, to this day, they have never met.

Stacey and Marlene

Stacey and I met at a little Greek restaurant in New York City, 54th and Madison. I had not seen the words egg cream used together in the same sentence in over forty years since I lived here, and have never been able to explain to anyone on the West Coast why this drink is called an egg cream. There is no egg. There is no cream. I ordered one, along with an egg salad sandwich on white. I was hoping the bread would be similar to the soft, squishy Wonder Bread of my youth. The same as I would order from that Bronx luncheonette on the days I would cut school so many years ago.

It was at this restaurant that Stacey and I shared family secrets, the secrets concerning Lorraine, our older sister. The sister that Stacey had essentially never met. The only connection she has is the baby book Lorraine bought to chronicle her birth and growth. At the time, Lorraine had every intention of watching Stacey grow through childhood. Lorraine was seventeen years old the year Stacey was born, and I was sixteen.

Stacey is a photographer. She received her MFA in Photography from CalArts. She has created a photo series journaling our older sister's suicide as a way to understand and connect with this unknown sibling, to calm some of the anxieties of growing up, of never knowing or even being told about Lorraine, only of her death from some mysterious disease that she might contract herself.

Closure was what she was looking for.

Stacey embarked on the project, compiling a series of photographs depicting, as she imagined, the events leading up to Lorraine's suicide.

Using her friends as models, she photographed them in poses with expressions of despair, loneliness, angst, and confusion. As part of the project, she discovered, and later visited the building where the suicide occurred. The address was published in a 1967 newspaper article.

The scene: an apartment building in Washington Square, Greenwich Village. Lorraine had been hospitalized at the time. The diagnosis was schizophrenia. It was then that I told Stacey my own little family secret: that Lorraine had called me the week before and told me she planned to kill herself. Unfortunately, I had never thought to tell anyone else. I didn't tell my parents what my sister had told me. At the time, I felt that I had handled it. My father was just recently home from the hospital himself after another manic-depressive episode, and Mom, well, didn't she have enough to deal with? I rode the wave of guilt, but now I realize it would not have changed anything.

Stacey and I were going to that building in Washington Square the next day. I expected it to be my most emotional experience on this trip. But the story I heard from Stacey in that Greek restaurant affected me even more. As part of her project in 1993, Stacey had already visited the building.

She told the doorman about her quest. The doorman remembered! He had heard the story from a colleague who was on duty that fateful day in October of 1967 when my sister ended her life.

The legend had lived on for thirty years.

Let me explain what I recall from fifty years ago. I was never told the details. I suppose my parents didn't even know. It was my Uncle Stan who had the grim task of journeying downtown to identify the body. My father, having been recently released from the hospital himself, was most likely in no shape, and my mother? No, my mother would not have gone. I knew how troubled Lorraine was, and since she had told me she was suicidal, this is the story I carried in my mind all these years:

She calmly walked into this building, got on the elevator, and went to the roof. She stood out on the top, contemplated, then made her decision. A decision that would quiet the demons in her head. A very calculated and calm decision and act.

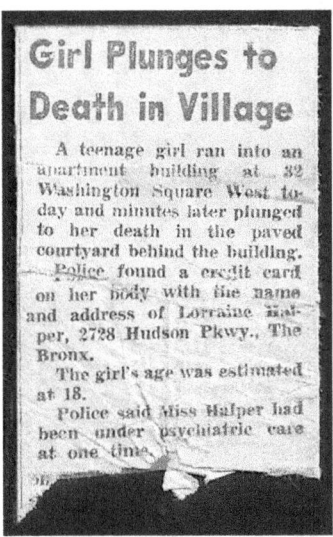

Girl Plunges to Death in Village

A teenage girl ran into an apartment building at 32 Washington Square West today and minutes later plunged to her death in the paved courtyard behind the building.

Police found a credit card on her body with the name and address of Lorraine Halper, 2728 Hudson Pkwy., The Bronx.

The girl's age was estimated at 18.

Police said Miss Halper had been under psychiatric care at one time.

My mind would not go further than this, and that was okay.

The story the doorman told my sister in 1993 differed greatly from the one I had conjured. He told Stacey that this girl came running into the building—hysterically screaming at the top of her lungs. She ran up one staircase as fast as she could. There were two staircases, one to the right and one to the left. As she ran up the left staircase, the doorman ran up the right, trying to catch her, trying to stop her—but he said he could not believe how fast she was. She made it to the landing of the sixth floor and, without pausing, went right out the open window.

This was very different than my self-created memory of a calm and contemplated decision, a very calculated, almost peaceful act.

Now the truth was before me: violent and horrifying, done in wrenching misery, panic, anguish, hopelessness. I cried that day in that Greek restaurant. I cried for the violence, for the senselessness, and I cried for mental illness.

When we finally went to the building in Washington Square the next day, I was ready.

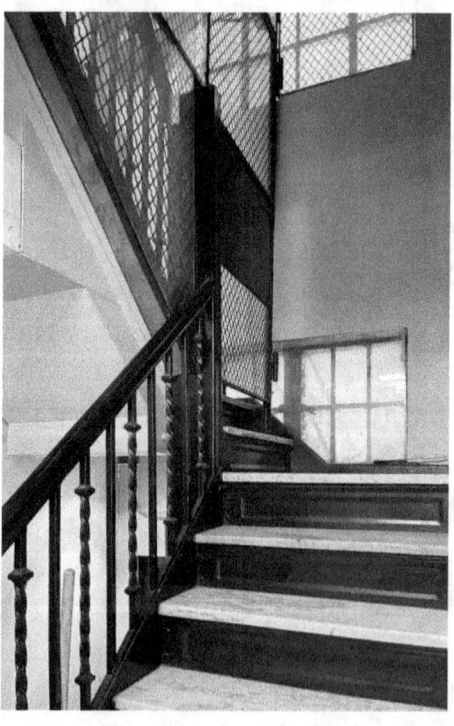

There was a gate closing off the stairway to the left. We did not say who we were or why we were there, but when we asked about the gates across the staircase, according to building legend, the current doorman told us that a long time ago, a girl ran up those stairs and jumped out a window. There has been a gate there ever since.

To the best of my knowledge, neither Stacey nor I have ever told our parents the truth of what we learned had happened on that dreadful day in Washington Square. Our parents are gone now. I suppose now, we, too, are keeping family secrets.

~~

Why 32 Washington Square?

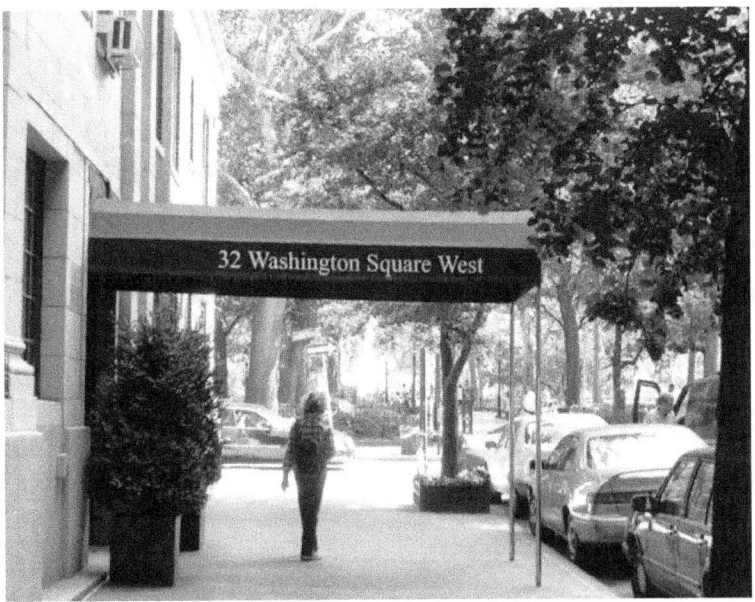

The question had always lingered: why that building? Why and how did she leave a hospital on Staten Island and travel the twenty miles or so by subway, bus, or ferry to that particular spot in Greenwich Village? I suspected her psychiatrist lived in that building or perhaps had his office there. She said she had been in love with the handsome doctor with the British accent, which is not at all unusual in a psychiatrist's life.

A few years back, I searched the internet for her doctor. I found him and wrote to him, asking some questions about my sister's condition and whether he was connected to that address. I never received an answer. But I was not surprised. I don't think I ever expected to.

My father was an avid sixteen-millimeter movie buff. He had his camera with him for every occasion, usually to the exasperation of the rest of the family. Every Halloween, my friends would groan as the door would open, and the lights would blind them. We did have the best treats in the building, so the kids would come. Every Christmas, a present could not be opened without being recorded. In the 1950s, he took my sisters and me down to that exact place. Washington Square Park, Greenwich Village, to record the antics of the beatniks who would hang out at the fountain and listen to the singers harmonizing in the echo under the Washington Square Arch. It was just across the street from 32 Washington Square West.

Claudia

There is an interesting family dynamic at play here. The two children most impacted at the time Dad started lithium in 1966 or 1967 would be my younger sister, Claudia, and me. She was twelve years old, and I was sixteen.

My sister would tell me that she grew up lacking love and attention from our parents. I can understand that. There was always so much drama. Dad was going in and out of hospitals. Lorraine was doing the same, with intermittent catatonia and psychosis that none of us understood at the time. Warren was born only eighteen months later than Claudia, and there was always anxiety and concern over him until and after he was placed in the first private institution at age three and a half. Always someone in crisis to take care of. It seemed that if we didn't have a problem in this family of dysfunction, we were left to our own devices. It had shaped her life and profoundly impacted her, even to this day, suffering severe panic attacks and rejection issues.

> The greatest terror a child can have is
> that he is not loved,
> and rejection is the hell he fears.
>
> ~John Steinbeck, *East of Eden*

Claudia comments: *In contrast, perhaps because I was a little older, my mantra has always been:*

As the middle child of a manic-depressive father and schizophrenic sister I was lucky enough to have been completely ignored. I consider myself one of the lucky ones.

At a time when a budding teenager certainly doesn't want or need overly attentive parents, I could come and go as I pleased. But I never felt unloved. I guess I didn't need that same attention, which allowed me to get away with a lot. No one was watching.

When asked about her earliest memory of growing up in our family, Claudia remembers playing in the sandbox with her brother Warren. Then, one day, he was gone. No explanation. He was no longer her playmate. Warren was three years old at the time. Claudia was five. Warren was moved to a private institution in Yonkers. Perhaps she thought, "Will I be next? Did I do something wrong?"

She always looked up to Lorraine, who was five years older. She says, "I wanted to be like her; I wanted to look like her." Claudia was thirteen years old when Lorraine died and was afraid that she too would become mentally ill, become schizophrenic, and take her own life. That's a lot of fear for a thirteen-year-old to carry around. I think that's when the panic attacks started. Alcohol was the only way she could function. But no one knew. She functioned very well. She hid it from us all.

Claudia has been severely agoraphobic all her life. Agoraphobia literally means fear of the marketplace, but it's a lot more complicated than that. It's a fear of being in situations where escape might be difficult, or help isn't available if things go wrong. That will trigger a panic attack. Therefore, afraid of having a panic attack, it gets harder and harder to go anywhere that you don't feel safe. Agoraphobia is actually being afraid to leave your safe surroundings.

Her first awareness of its existence was in third grade at about eight years old. A girl in her class died from a seizure over the weekend. No one ever told the kids what happened. No counselors came into the classroom to ease their little minds. Just 'she had a seizure and died.' So, the biggest fear that Claudia can remember at that age, of course, was having a seizure and dying.

Much like the story of Stacey being told that the girl in those pictures on the wall was her sister: "She got sick and died." Then, the fear sets in.

Claudia does say that she was always aware that she was different from other kids. She lived in fear daily but never told any of us—Mom or Dad or sisters. She would look at people walking their dogs or going to the mailbox and think, "I'll be normal like that one day." I never saw this. I wasn't aware. At that point, I had kind of dissociated from the whole family.

Her drinking started at age twelve. Her first drink was a quart bottle of Colt 45. The first few sips made her feel like she had just taken a tranquilizer. It became her medicine. With alcohol, she was able to relax and let go of some fears, at least for a little while. So, the older she got, the more she drank, even hiding alcohol in her high school locker. Unfortunately, the agoraphobia also got worse. The more panic, the more alcohol.

She almost died in 1980, going through withdrawal on Mom and Dad's couch. As was her way, Mom pretended nothing was wrong, and Dad gave her one of his tranquilizers, which didn't help at all. The next morning, our brother and her husband took her to a local free clinic, where they took one look at her and shot her up with 50mg of Librium. She went to rehab, then AA meetings, and got sober. She would speak at meetings, hospitals, and even prisons about alcoholism.

Bruce

Bruce, born 1961, writes:

There were loud and joyous parties. There were dinner table political debates and laughter. There was a lot of beautiful music. They loved the good music of the day. Tony Bennett and Barbara Streisand. My sisters also had parties where all the girls and boys danced to Motown records.

And there were fights. There were mood swings. There was confusion.

I felt betrayed.

I recall the many arguments. One that I can't forget is watching mom hurl a heavy ashtray at dad. It was so disturbing because even at the age of six or seven, I was wise enough to detect that it was done in the heat of passion and of hate ... between my parents.

One night, my mother came home so drunk. I had never seen a person drunk before. I didn't know what it was, but she was not the mother I had ever known, and it frightened me to the point that I started to cry.

Years later, when I reflected on that night, I understood why it was so scary. It was like seeing an alien. When she appeared before me in a sort of altered state of mind, it was very frightening. I'd never seen 'wasted' before.

The betrayal from my father didn't come in the way of hitting or physical abuse; it was emotional abuse. It was my father's broken promises. He would pick a fight with me just to get out of something he had promised to do with me or for me. He once gave away my dog to people who wound up abusing him, even though he once told me that his father had also given his dog away, and it was the worst feeling ever. He would lie to people right in front of me, which was all very confusing.

Even though my father would say that he detested cursing and bad manners, one day on the elevator, while talking to an unknown face, he cursed like a sailor; it was vulgar and scary. I had never heard this kind of talk from him before in my life. I was shocked. Who was this man? Burt was a bit of a rebel, too. He used to steal French fries off of a stranger's plate after they left the restaurant. We were mortified. He was a grifter. He broke the law many times—not sure why. The last one was the 'book caper' in Albuquerque when he almost went to jail for mail fraud.

I would be shipped off to Westport, Connecticut, to spend the summers with my aunt, uncle, and cousins. I loved it, but it was different, and they had stricter rules. When I was six years old, I went up there in the fall of that year— October, as my oldest sister had just died. I didn't exactly know what happened.

My aunt would say to me, 'You weren't nurtured properly.'

I was a bedwetter, and she would be angry with me. She probably saw my emotional problems, but I was unaware of them until I was much older.

Even so, I felt safe in my home in the Bronx. The radio blaring in the mornings, and my older sisters fighting over pantyhose. I liked the noise and the commotion. Lots of family around. But I remember having emotional problems at a very young age, separation anxiety, and screaming and clinging to Claudia when she would go off to school.

The same thing would happen when my parents went out.

We had a maid who took care of me, Rebecca. She must have heard me crying and didn't console me. I felt very alone and afraid. I did love Rebecca, who was like a surrogate mother but showed little emotion. But, oh, the things she must have seen and heard. I figured she must have needed employment; otherwise, who would stick around for that?

It wasn't all bad. There was laughter, parties, and good music on a classic-sounding stereo; trips to Jones Beach in the summer and getting to listen to the pop station on the radio on the way home.

I don't really remember much about Lorraine or Warren.

One afternoon, I came home from playing in the streets to find a houseful of people in the living room, including Father Boyle, the local priest. What was I told?

'Your sister died. She had an accident. She fell on her head.'

Something was off about the way this news was presented to me. I was confused and remember being angry because I didn't know how to respond. I was six years old. I said something like, 'Who cares?' or a similar cavalier comment. I still think about that reaction to this day. It would be another five years before I found out that 'falling on her head' meant that she purposely jumped off a building.

I only remember one car ride with our brother Warren. He was moved to an institution three years before I was even born.

We moved to Arizona when I was thirteen, and new schools once again. It was lonely. I was now a teenager and could see my father for the broken man he really is— broke and running from the bill collectors back in New York. We had a smaller apartment, and I was too close to the madness.

He did, however, support my musical dreams. I was into rock and roll. We'd have talks after I came home from recording with some older musicians in town. We did bond at times. But there was always a fight over money or something else.

There were things I loved about my dad. He was smart. Book smart and funny with a sort of wacky sense of humor. He was handsome, like Cary Grant; gregarious and a charmer, especially with the ladies. He loved the thrill of the hunt, landing a sale, closing a deal.

He loved music, especially good music: Mario Lanza, Tony Bennett, Barbara Streisand.

He had a rich and painful life in the best city in America— perhaps the world, with a cast full of characters. He was lonely and had few friends, if any. He got along well with women more. He was a feminist and a conversationalist.

Insecure, he tried to elevate himself above others to seem superior. He seemed to trick others with his fancy and practiced words to make them feel inferior.

Perhaps the greatest betrayal of all.

He would have loved show business. He should have been an actor. And, in a way, he was. He would often quote, 'All the world's a stage, and we are merely players' line, paraphrased.

I now realize that I identify with his manic side. An occasional euphoria about just being alive in the world. Then later in life, I would choose girlfriends who would also betray me.

I didn't call him out on his betrayals at the end when I went to see him on his deathbed at the VA hospital. What would be the point? I decided that I would sing to him instead, to tell him that I was going to sing like Tony Bennett. And that was my gift to him—To sing.

Maybe their love of music was their gift to me, after all.

In the end, I couldn't blame my father for his mental illness; it wasn't his fault.

It is our choice whether to hate something in our lives or to love every moment of them, even the parts that bring us pain.

At every moment, we are volunteers.

~Stephen Colbert (1)

Stacey

Stacey, born 1966, writes:

When I look back and think about my parents' behavior in those days, always keeping a watchful eye on me, they were probably looking for signs of schizophrenia by the age of twelve or so, when it can start to manifest. That watchful eye was only about their fears. They had no idea of the fears I was living with. They were otherwise somewhat hands-off as I grew up. Sports and good friends were more like family to me. They were dealing with their own issues. I kept my distance. My parents' relationship in those years was quite tense.

I am the youngest of six. Lorraine was the eldest, eighteen years older. I had worried for so many years that I might get sick and die for no apparent reason, and then when Claudia told me the whole story at fourteen or fifteen, I worried that I would become mentally ill. Other than those intense fears, I really did not think much about Lorraine. She was a stranger.

After I finished college in New York, I moved back to Tucson, and that is when I became very interested in Lorraine. What was she actually like? I suddenly could not stop thinking about her and wondering, was I like her? Did we share similar interests? I began inundating my poor mother with questions about Lorraine. My mother didn't really want to talk about her. My mother never wanted to talk about anything negative from the past that she had already buried. She lived in her own reality. One day, Mom walked out of the guest bedroom carrying a large cardboard box. She handed it to me and said, 'These are Lorraine's mementos, photographs, etc. You may have this. It will help you learn more about her.' I thanked her and then pored over the contents—This box of Lorraine—This box was Lorraine; it was a goldmine.

One of the most fascinating and sad items was my baby book, tracking my first year of life—a gift from Lorraine. After the first few months, the pages are all blank.

I finished studying Fine Art Photography in New York before returning to Tucson. A friend invited me to show my work in a gallery downtown. I jumped at the opportunity and immediately knew what I would show in that gallery space. Born was the idea for a series of sixteen small black and white images recreating, with my artist friends, the life of Lorraine up until her death (as I knew it). This is the artist's statement that went along with the presentation, followed by the photos themselves.

I recently located my baby book, a gift from Lorraine, given to me at birth. The book was meant to record the events of my first years of life. But only the first months were recorded. The stark emptiness of the book is representative of a twenty-six-year gap between that gift and this series of photographs. This series is a depiction of my thoughts about the last years of my sister's life. The images have come to me through letters and poetry left behind by Lorraine.

I studied them as an attempt to demystify her death, to make real her presence in my life.

This series is a gift to her.

I have chosen the palladium process to create these images because, being hand done, it allows more intimacy and involvement with the work. This process is one of the most archival photographic methods. My intention is to preserve and recognize the memory of Lorraine's life solidly. I do not want her to be forgotten or her memory to fade away.

The process of making those images and having a public showing was freeing. I felt the weight of Lorraine suddenly lifted. Catharsis at its finest.

The Lorraine Series

© Stacey Halper 1993

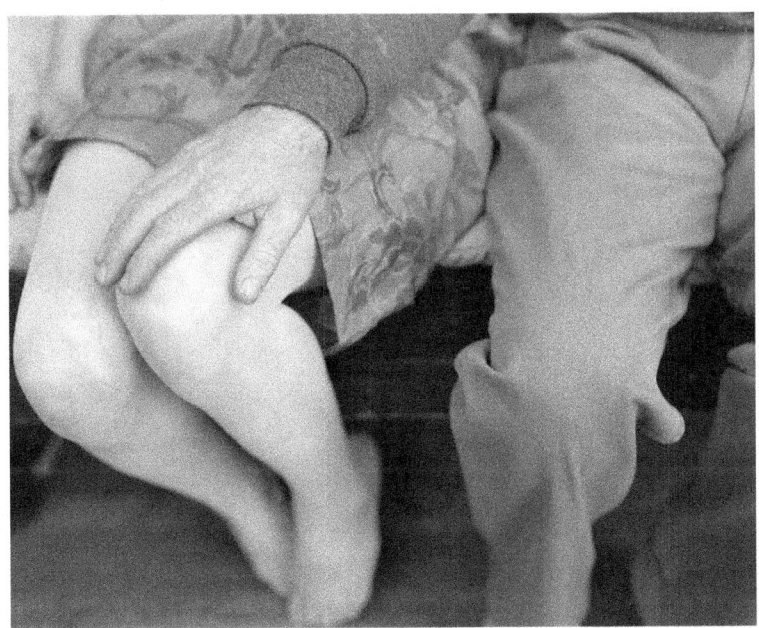

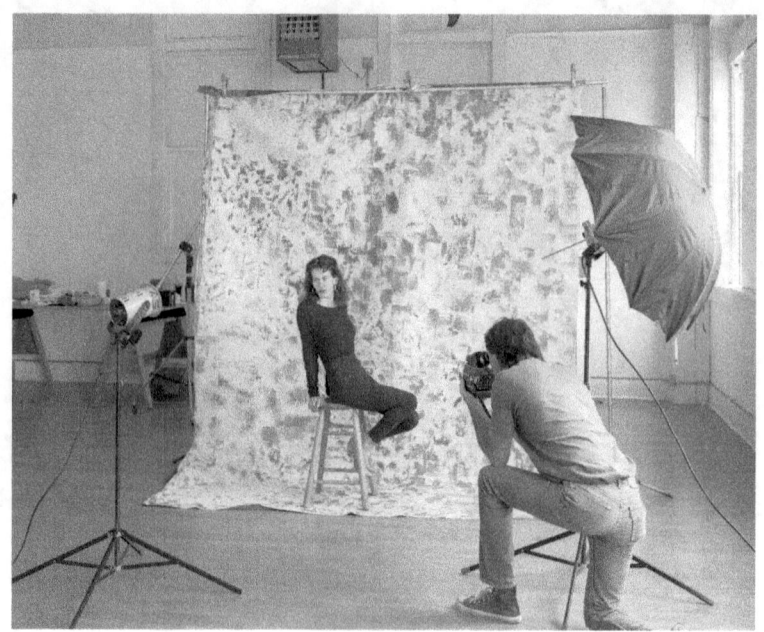

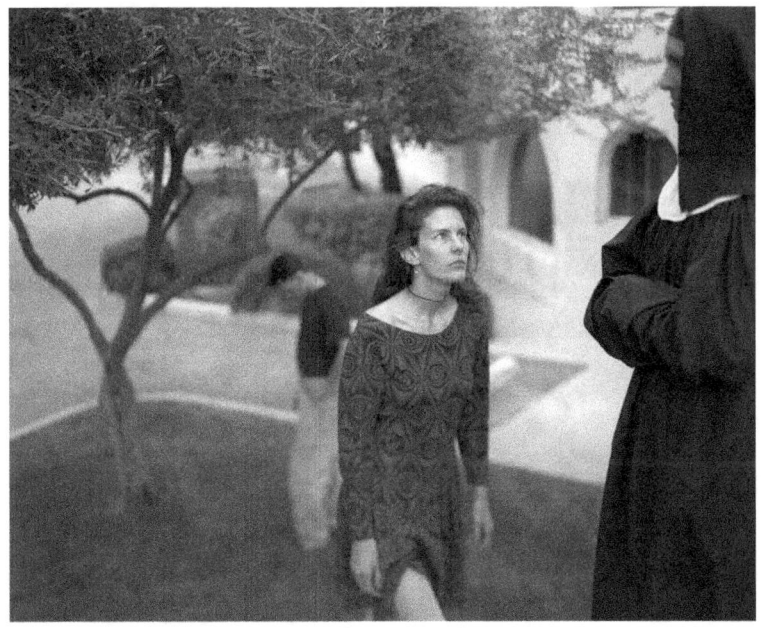

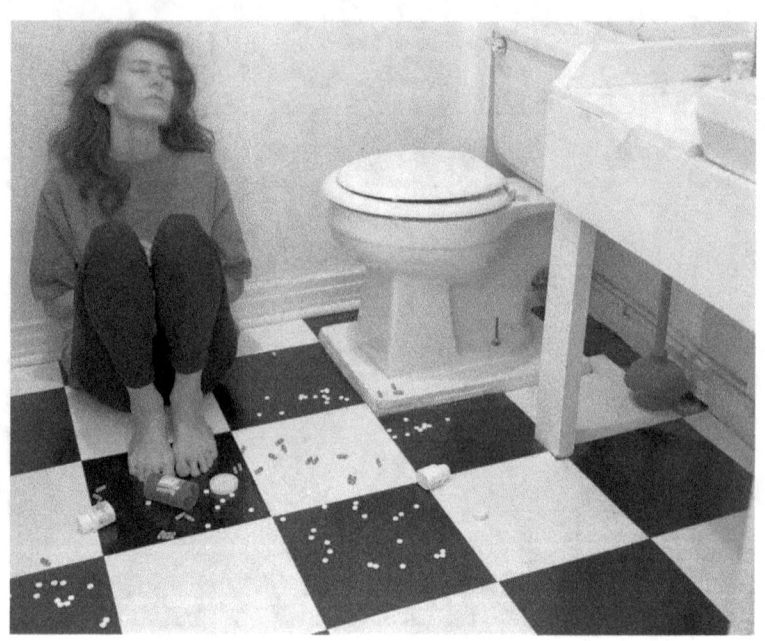

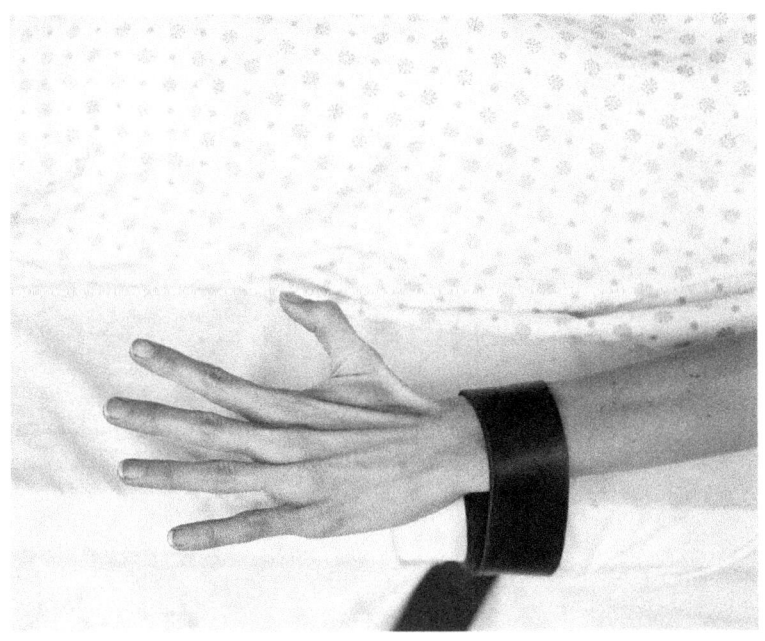

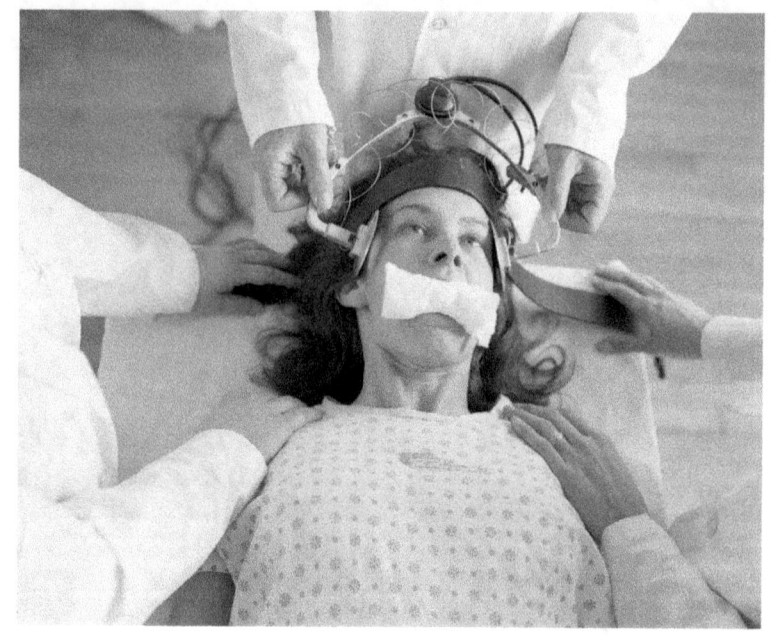

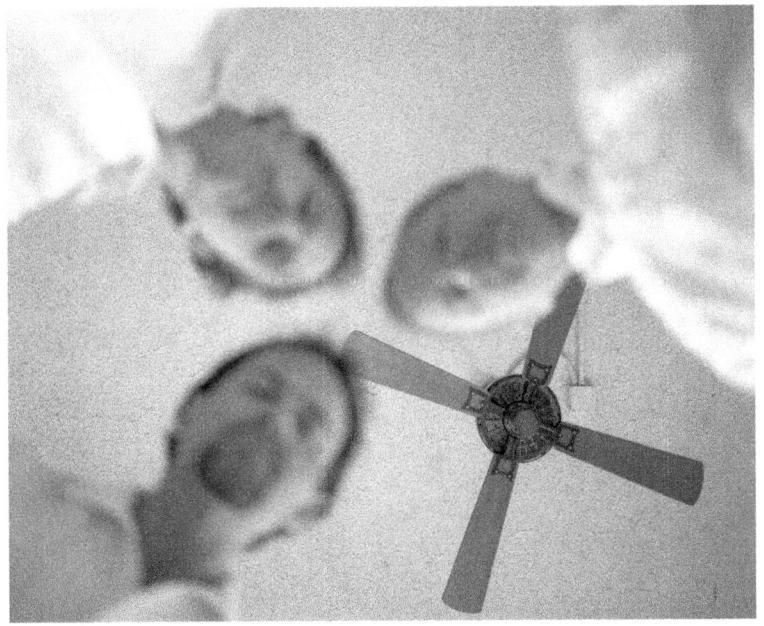

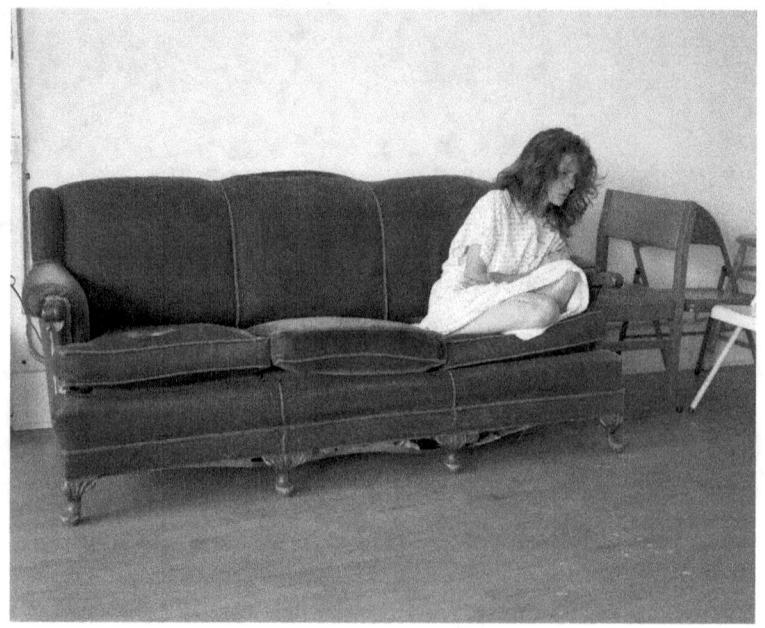

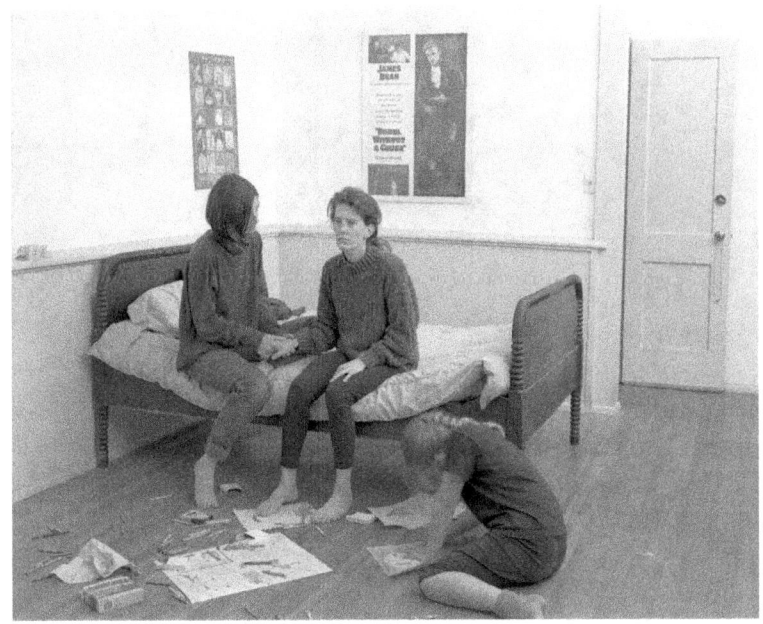

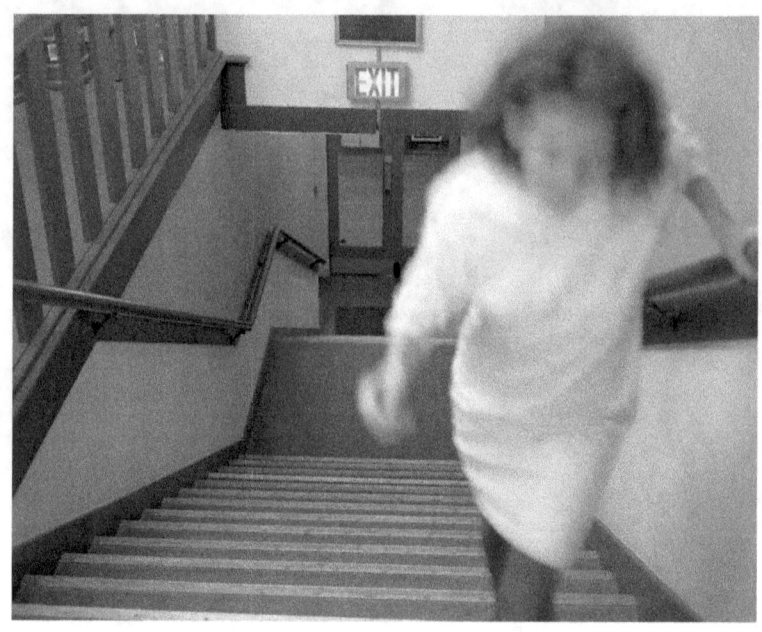

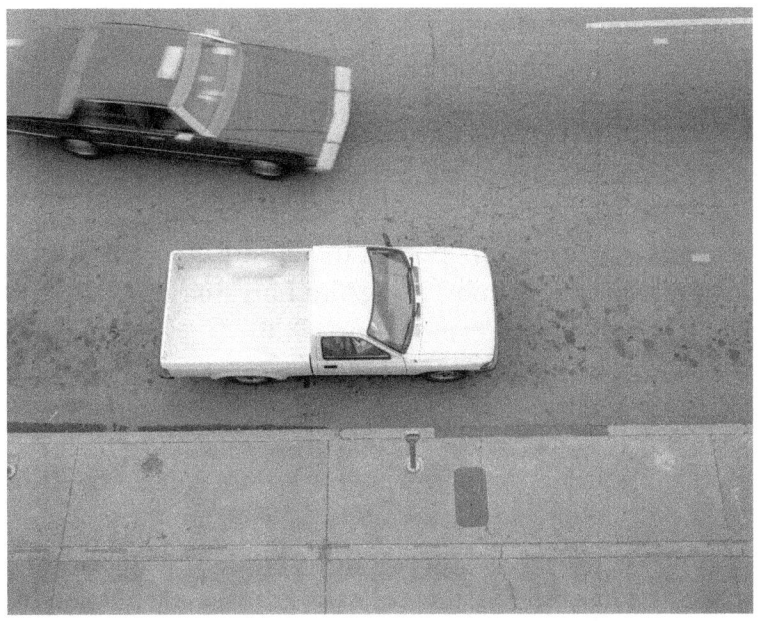

A Response to Stacey's Photos

Stacey's first picture (hand on knee) brings me to another Family Secret.

It had been alleged that my father had sexually abused my sister Lorraine in the past, but when in the past is unknown. The reason it has become a family story, a family secret, is because my father admitted to this act.

During one of his psychotic episodes at one of his many hospital stays, he confessed this story to his brother. His brother told his wife. His wife (our aunt) told my sister Stacey, and she carried it with her for years—she still does.

Since Stacey was not a part of the family dynamic during my and Lorraine's upbringing and Lorraine and I were so close in age, Stacey came to me with the question. What did I think of this rumored family secret?

Remember the story of my dad stabbing himself in the stomach during a psychotic episode that committed him to Bellevue for six months of his life? That is the logic I used with Stacey and also the logic I have used with myself. If he could falsely believe that he was the man on TV and go to the extremes that he did—he was also capable of telling his brother this disturbing story—it didn't necessarily mean it was true. Both my sisters believe it is true.

Unfortunately, we will never know.

Lorraine's Friends

I contacted a few of Lorraine's friends from our grade school. The neighborhood Catholic school was where we all went from kindergarten to eighth grade. We all lived in close proximity, in apartment buildings and on neighborhood streets. We knew each other's friends, and it seemed everyone had a sibling a grade ahead or a grade behind.

In the age of Facebook, I found a few of them, some still actually living in Riverdale. One friend said that no one in their group knew she was ill. She was different but sweet and always smiling. After eighth grade graduation, Lorraine went away to boarding school, and the next thing they knew, she committed suicide. Another friend who grew up in the building with us said she seemed very sad around sixth grade, age twelve. Other than that, nothing seemed out of the ordinary to them. No one knew she had been hospitalized. No one knew she was schizophrenic. All they knew was, one day in October of 1967, they were told that she had committed suicide. And they were shocked.

There was a stigma around mental illness in 1967. Of course, there still is today, but I do think we have come a long way. Statistics show that to be true.

Mom and Dad

Mom and Dad always had a pretty rocky relationship. There were summers when Dad would pack up his brown wooden boxes of Oneida silverware and take the show on the road. Sometimes, we would also go along. There were also times when he went by himself. He had a favorite place in Connecticut, The Old Saybrook Inn. Later in life, I found out he was having an affair with someone at the Inn. That is probably why it was his favorite place. I wasn't surprised. I always suspected there were probably more affairs. He was quite suave, good-looking, and loved to flirt. When manic, he could take on the world.

A memory that I have never been able to shake is of driving somewhere, I don't remember where, with the whole family in the car – whoever that consisted of at the time. I had recently gotten my driver's license so it must have been about 1966 or 1967, just around the time Dad started taking lithium. I would guess it was more like valium than lithium in his system because when I looked over at him, driving down the highway, his eyes were closed. Closed! I yelled. His eyes opened and I made him pull off the road. To my surprise he did and I got behind the wheel and drove the rest of the way home. That incident shook me to the core. The thought of what could have happened.

I don't talk much about Mom during those days. I gave you her history and how she and my father met. I'm sure she didn't realize the trickery involved in that union for years. Or maybe she did. Perhaps her desire for the good life outweighed the yet-unknown life. As I got to know her friends in Tucson during her later years, it seems that all they really knew of Joan was the privileged life she led in New York City. Dinners at Tavern on the Green and Broadway shows. It was easier to dine out, as she would phrase it, on stories of grandeur rather than devastation and loss. She didn't talk very much about the tragedies of her life. She didn't want to think about it. My mother was very caring but did not show her emotions in the physical huggy/kissy kind of way. I always, however, felt loved by her. She would tell her friends about how well I was doing in school, how I was such a help with the family situations, or whatever endeavor I took on—my mother would always praise me. Her bragging embarrassed me, as I certainly didn't feel I deserved it. I feel that she decided to focus on me rather than what was really going on around her.

Mom didn't lose her temper with the kids very often, but she did with Dad. I remember one dinner when Mom had enough of whatever my father was spewing, and she methodically turned over every plate of spaghetti on the table. Sauce and pasta splashed all over the floor and walls. I'm not sure how old I was, but it was scary—at any age. Bruce says he remembers running from the dining room to be comforted by me—but I just laughed it off. That's how I expressed my emotions and still do to some degree today. I'm sure I was just as scared and upset about the scene as everyone else was.

Mom would cope by drinking. After one of these episodes, she would go over to a friend's apartment to cool off. Theresa was next door. Her best friend and drinking buddy, Dee, was on the fourth floor. They would drink their scotch and try to forget. Hudson Gardens was like a small town.

Dad would always tell us kids that mom was an alcoholic. I don't remember ever seeing her out of control, in contrast to the story my brother tells of seeing her wasted. But that may have been just a difference in our ages (eleven years) and how young he was when having that memory and how much older I was. Maybe her drinking did get worse, or maybe I was just not paying attention. One thing I know is that miraculously, after my parent's divorce around the late nineteen-eighties, Mom stopped drinking. I know there is a very strong connection between bipolar disorder and alcoholism. Thankfully, Dad never drank.

I have always assumed that Claudia's agoraphobia and maybe even Stacey's panic attacks had come from my mother's set of genes rather than my father's. As Mom got older it was harder and harder for her to leave the house. The fact that she didn't drive and that where we lived in New York, everything from dry cleaning to alcohol could be delivered straight to your door, didn't encourage her to leave. I remember a story when my kids were young and she was visiting. We went to a school play. Mom needed to sit in the back of the auditorium and on the end of the aisle. I suppose this was to be able to get out fast. Well, as the auditorium was filling up, chairs kept being added to the end of the row. Mom would have to get up and move to the new end of the row. Then more chairs were added and Mom would have to move to the new end of the row again. You get the picture. To me it was funny, but I'm sure to Mom it was terrifying.

Following are a couple of short stories I wrote about my dad. True stories—interesting and sad.

My Dad, the Imposter

I am unsure about the timing, whether before or after lithium, but Dad would go to his weekly group therapy at the VA Hospital in New York. The story goes that the therapist leading the group had to quit for some reason, and Dad took over the group. He assured everyone that it was okay; he was a therapist—not sure if he actually used the word licensed. This went on for quite a while until someone figured it out. Not only was he fired from his fake leadership position, but he was also asked to leave therapy altogether.

When I told this story to my sister, she said, "Oh, yeah, he used to tell people all the time that he was a therapist." She remembers going up the elevator to our apartment one day, and he was telling the other passengers that he was a therapist.

My brother recounts a similar story. He remembered being so confused one day when he heard my father telling someone on the elevator that he was a doctor, or a psychologist, or something untrue. He was only a six-year-old boy, but he knew his father was a salesman.

A few years ago, I got a message on Facebook from someone who recognized my name. "Is Burt your father?" she asked. When I told her he was, she went on to tell me how grateful she and her whole family were to my father. "He saved my mother's life. He was her sponsor at AA, and she always credited him with her sobriety." That was a nice story, except for the fact that my father did not drink. Dad going to AA? Not because he was an alcoholic that's for sure. My conclusion was the therapist syndrome again. He loved to be the hero in his own story. Or maybe just an affair.

My Dad and the Book Caper

One of my dad's passions was buying and selling antiques. He had a real knack for that and became quite knowledgeable. Being a peddler in New York City and working on his own schedule gave him the time to pursue this interest. Being the great salesman that he was worked in his favor, too, when bartering for items of interest. It was a never-ending surprise, coming home from school to see which pieces of art were missing from the apartment walls and what beautiful porcelain pieces were added to the collection in the breakfront. Mom had to sometimes throw her body on top of a piece she loved so it would not be re-sold.

Dad's illustrious sales career ended in 1974 with the advent of credit cards and discount stores. Direct and door-to-door sales became a thing of the past.

He had been taking lithium and had remained relatively stable. He decided to move the family, or what was left of the family, to Tucson, Arizona. There were only my youngest brother and sister still living at home. My sister Claudia and I were old enough to have escaped (ahem ... that is) left home by this time.

One theory was that Dad was running away from the creditors. He owed money all over town. Another was that he was filled with guilt at not being able to continue to pay for the private facility my brother lived in and had to be sent to Willowbrook.

By moving the family 2,000 miles away, he would not have to visit. There was, perhaps, truth to both theories. Dad had fond memories of having lived in Tucson after being discharged from the Army in 1946 for health reasons.

Things did not go well for Dad in Tucson, which is another chapter altogether. He and Mom divorced after thirty-six years. He immediately found someone else (no comment) who adored him (he loved to be adored); he remarried and moved to Albuquerque.

When in Albuquerque, he discovered the flea market. Dad would find collectibles, antiques, and paintings like he did in New York and barter, feigning naïveté when he knew what a bargain would be had. He would set up his tables every weekend and prominently display a picture frame with a price tag of $10,000. Of course, anyone who saw it would wonder how that empty picture frame could be worth $10,000. It started many a conversation and sold many pieces of his wares. The picture frame was worth $2.00.

Dad ... Priceless!

But he wanted to do something different.

He was buying from his fellow flea marketers and then re-selling the same wares at a much higher price. This did not gain him the title of Mr. Congeniality.

He remembered a time when he was in high school, he ordered books from book clubs to build up his library but never paid for them. He would get letters with threats of collection and lawsuits but realized that the cost of litigation for these companies would be more than they would collect. He ignored them, and soon, the letters and threats stopped coming. "Why not do that again?" he thought. The plan was hatched.

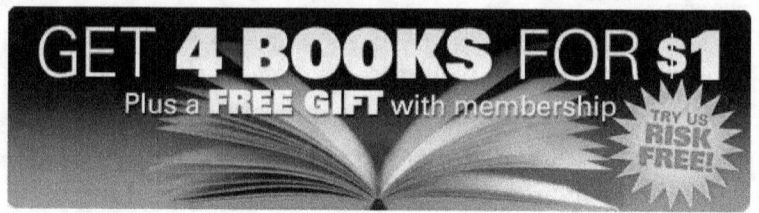

He opened dozens of post office boxes all over town with fictitious names. I know this because I went to visit one fall, and during a tour of the town, Dad said he had a few stops to make along the way. He pulled up to at least six or seven mail drops, those private post-office box companies with names like Mail Post or Postal Depot, Mail Boxes, Etc., etc. While he was picking up his mail at one of his drops, I took a peek in the back seat of his Toyota hatchback. There were envelopes five inches deep. It looked like junk mail. I started sifting through, and sure enough, there was envelope after envelope from publishing house after publishing house in the names of: *Oh my god, there is the name of my uncle*, who died in 1979; Our next-door neighbor in the Bronx, who died in 1967. There were many other names recognizable to me of deceased relatives and friends. There was even an envelope addressed to my dead sister. What was going on?

When Dad returned to the car, I confronted him, told him what I had discovered, and demanded to know what was happening. He replied that he did not want me to be involved, so he would not tell me but assured me that what he was doing was not illegal. There was no sense arguing with my dad.

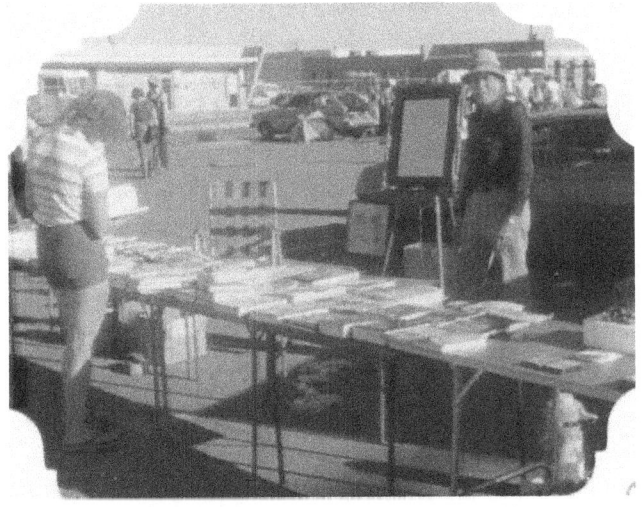

That's Dad with the hat, selling his contraband, standing next to a blank picture frame priced at $10,000 (his gimmick to draw attention and start a conversation).

About six months later, there was a knock at his door. Federal marshals. He was under arrest. My Dad was arrested for mail fraud, a federal offense and a felony that could bring up to five years of jail time and a $25,000 fine for "using a fictitious name or address in a fraudulent activity."

One of his flea market brethren and competition had turned him in. Apparently, this fellow could not imagine how Dad could be selling brand-new hardback books, CDs, and tapes for three and four dollars apiece.

Even at 1986 prices, this was a steal. (No pun intended). He would bring home up to $400 a weekend from the flea market, so you can imagine how many books he had. I don't suppose it could have lasted too much longer anyway.

He went to trial. He was scared to death, to say the least, and was put on probation for five years and had to pay back, I believe, $5,000. He learned his lesson well. But up until the day he died, he would reiterate the statement: "I knew what I was doing was immoral, but I had no idea it was illegal."

Marlene

(That's me), born 1950.

A friend who read my manuscript raised the question of why I tell of my siblings' memories and reactions but do not talk much about my own. My answer was that I don't have a lot of memories but I'll give it a try.

As I have said, I always felt loved by my mother. As far as my father was concerned, I guess I always assumed he loved me and the rest of his children. I think I was always cognizant, to some extent, that what was going on with my father was somehow not his fault and my mother's apparent emotional distance was her way of coping with her own challenges. She had a lot of coping to do.

To this day, I am not a very emotional person. I often wonder if it is because I had to keep my emotions deep inside in order not to be another family problem. I was the one in the family, whether due to age or mental capacity, that was counted on. Between my mom and me, we organized that move from the two-apartment setup back to Hudson Gardens when Dad was hospitalized at the same time Lorraine was hospitalized.

Mom never had a driver's license. She never drove a car, so those last few years between my sister's hospitalizations and death, I was also the taxi driver, the grocery shopper, and whatever else that needed being done, while also finding time to hang out and smoke pot with my friends in the park. I was sixteen years old in 1966, the year I got my driver's license and also started smoking pot. Seems I have always been good at multitasking.

I had a bad case of mononucleosis when I was sixteen. Doctor said 'no alcohol' for six months. Not sure how the doctor knew I drank alcohol but nevertheless, I sought out those few friends who I knew were smoking pot. Not only was it illegal in 1966, of course, but also not cool. My friends, especially the Irish Catholics, thought only hippie types did stuff like that.

It is said that the feelings you had to hide as a child are still within you. Suppressed emotions or repressed? Suppression is simply shutting down. You push those emotions out of your consciousness because you don't know what to do with them or simply don't want to deal with them. It allows a person to avoid uncomfortable feelings. If you avoid them, you think you can forget them and in turn, don't have to deal with them. If you don't feel your emotions, they can't hurt you. The reality of it though is that they never disappear and they will eventually affect us all in different ways.

This path leaves you feeling kind of numb. Drinking scotch on the rocks every night will also make you feel numb. This sounds like my mother. She did not lack compassion but I think she had suppressed so much emotion over the years that, well, it just left her numb. But can I blame her?

Whereas repressing those feelings is more of an unconscious defense mechanism to avoid them. A coping mechanism. Repression of memories may happen because an individual dissociates themselves while undergoing trauma, to be able to survive through it. The latter sounds more like me.

It's been an interesting endeavor to try and tie the past to the choices I made in life. The partner I eventually married, for example. They say that some people tend to marry a person similar to one of their parents. The theory is based on the idea that we are trying to unconsciously resolve parental conflict. It feels familiar and it keeps us in that cycle of dysfunction. I certainly did that. Another major choice in my life was to join a cult.

~~

In my early twenties, I would become involved with a right-wing fundamentalist Christian group, which I now call a cult. Of course, at the time, that was the farthest thing from my mind. As they say, "No one *joins* a cult." You wake up one day, sometimes years later, to see it for what it really is. It is a very slow indoctrination and manipulation. In my case, I woke up fifteen years later.

When you bring up the fact you were in a cult, people immediately think of Jonestown, Charlie Manson, The Moonies. It wasn't as extreme as that, but there is a spectrum. In the end, if you are manipulated to believe what the group believes, without question, you are probably in a cult. If you question the doctrine or teaching, then something must be wrong with you. If you keep questioning, you will probably be ostracized. And, if ostracized, it will be said you are of the devil. My cult was started by a man who says that God audibly told him he would teach him the Word (the Bible) as it had not been taught since the first-century church if he would teach it to others. We were the chosen ones, so to speak, to sit at his feet, to learn that Word he was teaching us. We were special. (Red flag!) The 'Teacher' said the original language of the Bible was Aramaic which was then translated to Greek which was then translated to German, then to English. Therefore, he had to tell us what the real translation was. I didn't speak Aramaic, or Greek, or German. I thought he must have known what he was talking about. (Another one of those pesky red flags). What the Teacher really did was interpret the Scriptures to fit his own theological position. When he needed to, he could twist the Greek and Hebrew words to mean what he wanted. The Teacher was very good at making the Bible say what he wanted it to say, just as every other false teacher does.

It was the early seventies. There was the constant stream of cocaine and marijuana to keep us all nourished, with the right amount of rock-n-roll and long-haired musicians stirred in to create the perfect mix. Sex, drugs, and rock-n-roll! Those were the days. Those were also the days of taking a long, hard look at what the future would hold. I was heading quickly toward adulthood and didn't have a working compass. Though a college dropout, I was smart enough to realize that this lifestyle had a relatively short shelf life. In hindsight, I can see that the drugs and promiscuity came from a need to be wanted. To be seen. To be loved.

The Jesus Freak movement started in San Francisco and rapidly moved across the United States. There were no people in orange robes or shaved heads. We were all counterculture ex-hippie types looking for the same thing.

In the May 14, 1971 edition of *Life* magazine, there was an article called The Groovy Christians of Rye, New York:

Youngsters Go on a Religion Trip and Leave Many Parents Baffled. They were bewildered because their children had become Christians. That was the group I had joined, The Way, and I went to those meetings in Rye, New York, only about fifteen miles from where I lived. I then traveled around the country for three years, spreading the word. Independence, Missouri; New Bedford, Massachusetts; and Seattle, where I met my future husband, who was also in the group, of course, and settled down.

I would never in a million years have believed that someone could so convince me to be a blind follower of anything, without question, without doubt. Oh, there were questions, and there was doubt. Still, the love, the absolute acceptance in the group, gradually and almost without notice, became my entire life. I was manipulated to believe that I had made my own decision.

> Most citizens like to think that their own minds and thought processes are invulnerable. 'Other people can be manipulated, but not me,' they declare.
>
> ~ Margaret Singer, Ph.D.

Since most of us didn't know anything about the Bible to begin with—the Catholic church certainly didn't teach us the Bible—and the fact that some of the fabulous things this dynamic teacher was teaching just happened to be at cross purposes with organized religion, was even better. As a culture, in the early 1970s, we were pretty much against anything organized. Yes, I now realize I had just jumped from one organized system to another.

None of us started out wanting to join a cult. We wanted to join a movement. We wanted to help people, we wanted to change the world, be part of something bigger than ourself. The perfect storm, as they say, is a person who is seeking, who is open-minded, looking for answers, and then you run into someone who says they have the answers. "Oh my!" you think, "God must have sent these people to me." Then there is the love bombing. You show up at a meeting, a Bible study, a fellowship, whatever they call it, and everybody is so overly friendly. They want to hug you, say God bless you, or whatever their own vernacular is. Now I know that when you feel too good too fast—that's a red flag!

I never had much of a father figure to look up to. Was that why I was now looking to God? Was the love I felt in that Bible study room what I had longed for all my life?

After some weeks, I decided that cleaning up my life a bit wouldn't be a bad thing. My joining this group changed the course of my life from drugs and promiscuity to the Bible. That was a good thing. In hindsight, however, I can also see that what it did was take away from me something huge: The ability to think for myself. The ability to question or doubt; to trust myself. I put all my trust in a person, not God, even though it was made to look that way.

The fact that my marriage was bad from the start didn't help matters. It seems I had found the dysfunction I grew up with and married him. We were taught to believe that any two believers could marry and be compatible, because they both had the Lord in their lives. Divorce was definitely frowned upon. Breaking a commitment like that (made before God) would not only ostracize me from the group, my friends, but I would be walking away from God. After fourteen years, I was indoctrinated enough to believe that if I strayed away from the group and didn't adhere to its teachings and beliefs, I would be fodder for the devil, as they put it. Had they told me this the first day I went to the Bible study with my friend Ellen, I would have run in the other direction as fast as I could. No, it was a very slow process, this indoctrination.

It's been a long, strange road, to be sure, but I take full responsibility for my decisions. I made the decision to continue going back to the fellowship meetings, take the classes, and marry the man I married. I learned a lot along the way. Perhaps the biggest thing I learned was to think for myself, and if it took fifteen years for that, well, that's okay. Some people never learn.

I was always *so* proud of myself for not being mentally ill in my mentally ill family that I denied for a long time that The Way was a cult, as that would make me less of a strong, independent person.

Strong and mentally balanced individuals ... do not join cults!

MARLENE DUNHAM

PART 5 – THE DNA CONNECTION

MARLENE DUNHAM

Autism

I have always wondered whether my father's diagnosis and my sister's diagnosis could have been the same. Both had psychotic incidents and delusions. And one day, I wondered about my brother Warren. What if he were autistic? What if he had never been institutionalized at age three and a half.

He spent the next twenty-seven years in institutions, fifteen of those years at Willowbrook. What if? What if?

According to Very Well Health.com (1), The most severe type of autism, also known as level three, presents itself with the following:

1. Nonverbal or very limited speech

2. Sensory processing issues—sensory overload

3. Extreme difficulty with changes in routine

4. Behavioral challenges, i.e., aggression, wandering, or running away

5. Self-injury—head banging, violent rocking back and forth

6. Pica—eating non-food items

7. Repetitive behaviors and self-stimulatory behaviors

All of the above are behaviors that my brother has exhibited, although, to my knowledge, he has never been diagnosed with level three autism. His original diagnosis was severe mental retardation. His more recent diagnosis (2002) from Sunmount Developmental Center:

- Infantile autism active state

- Seizure disorder

- Organic brain syndrome

- Pica

It was said that Warren was 'selectively mute.' What if he were taught to speak? He could speak; he had a voice because he would parrot words when he was a toddler at home. Echolalia is a behavior where a person repeats words or phrases they've heard, often as a way of communication or self-stimulation. He just would not or could not form words or sentences on his own. As Dr. Wilkins said in the previous interview:

These people were brought to Willowbrook to die there ... most of the time, they would stay there without going to school, without training, just rocking in a big empty room surrounded by other mentally retarded people.

It wasn't a school at all. Their life is just hours and hours of endless nothing to do.

He was treated as if he were mentally retarded. Was he?

Bipolar Disorder and Schizophrenia

These mental health conditions have some common traits and key differences. Even today, when the drug of choice, lithium, works on an individual, manic depression (better known today as Bipolar 1) is diagnosed. If lithium does not work, it would be on to another diagnosis. If a psychotic event is present, the patient would most likely be diagnosed as schizophrenic.

My family members were diagnosed over fifty years ago. Would either of their diagnoses be different today? Would it make any difference? I suppose it would make a difference in my family history and the genetic implications of passing down those genes.

Bipolar disorder causes shifts in mood, energy level, and thinking. Schizophrenia causes a person to appear to lose touch with reality. People with bipolar disorder may experience episodes of mania, often with periods of relative stability occurring in between. Individuals with schizophrenia experience symptoms of psychosis, such as hallucinations or delusions. (2) My father and my sister both had psychosis. Both had depression. Because of the overlap in symptoms, getting the proper diagnosis can be challenging. Also, a person can have both schizophrenia and bipolar disorder, which can complicate diagnosis. Some people have schizoaffective disorder, which involves a combination of schizophrenia symptoms and mood disorder symptoms. (2)

Quoting from the book entitled, *Lithium, It's Role in Psychiatric Research & Treatment,* by Samuel Gershon and Baron Shopsin:

The most difficult clinical problem is the separation of the manic patients from those with schizo-affective disorders.

They go on to say:

One reason why many schizophrenics have been studied in lithium trials is that their affective behavior may resemble that seen in the manic patients. (3)

They also note that there have been a significant number of reclassified diagnoses, from manic depressive to schizophrenic or schizo-affective. Those genetic implications were one of the reasons I had no children of my own until the age of thirty-seven, when the alarm on my biological clock started ringing in my ears. I rethought my decision, and by the age of thirty-nine, with the birth of twins, there were three. I've said that one of the things I am most grateful for is that it didn't stop me from having my three precious girls. And, as of this writing, three beautiful grandchildren. I'm certain that Dad never thought of great-grandchildren bouncing on his knee.

The Overlap

I recently came across an article on *Genetic Overlap between Autism, Schizophrenia, and Bipolar Disorder* by Liam S. Carroll and Michael J. Owen. (1)

The title certainly got my attention. Three members of my family suffered from these three apparently different disorders. I wondered for many years if there was a connection.

Carroll and Owen say that there is strong evidence that genetic factors make substantial contributions to the cause of autism, schizophrenia, and bipolar disorders, and they estimate that the inheritance factor could be upwards of 80%. It is a pretty well accepted fact that psychiatric disorders cluster in families and the evidence for a substantial role for genetic factors is undeniable. Even though traditionally considered separate diseases, this view has been challenged, (2) and a recent large-scale study has shown that relatives of individuals affected with schizophrenia have increased risks of bipolar disorder, and vice versa. (3)

Dr. Osman Shabir, a Postdoctoral Research Associate at the University of Sheffield, states:

Many mutations, polymorphisms and epigenetic changes that occur in Autism Spectrum Disorder, also occur in bipolar disorder and schizophrenia as well as other mental disorders (cross disorder association). (5)

There was my answer. The bipolar disorder of my father, schizophrenia of my sister, autism of my brother, and perhaps even the severe agoraphobia and panic attacks of my other sisters all had some sort of DNA connection. Of course, knowing this doesn't change anything, but maybe there is hope for the future—hope of earlier diagnosis, earlier interventions, and drugs to target specific genes. It satiated my wondering.

Epigenetics and Generational Trauma

Then, there is the conversation of generational trauma. It all gets so complex. This is a field of study that has been very controversial. I find it quite interesting and perhaps hopeful for future diagnoses and interventions. In a recent article by A. Abbas Naqvi, (1) he states that there seems to be an actual biological link bridging the gap between intergenerational trauma and the hard sciences. Epigenetics is an emerging field which investigates how:

... deeply social turmoil can impact populations and their descendants and environmental factors can affect genetic expression.

Epigenetics means on top of, or in addition to, genetics.

Evidence shows that communities that have suffered from trauma and persecution, i.e., Holocaust survivors and war veterans, can experience genetic changes that can then be transmitted to future generations. These changes affect our DNA but do not change its actual composition. (2)

One way that trauma passes down through generations is through epigenetic changes. The theory is that trauma changes how your genes work. Then, those changes pass down to your children. (3)

Rachel Yehuda, professor of psychiatry and Director of Traumatic Stress Studies Division at Mount Sinai, found that male Holocaust survivors who suffered from PTSD had children with lower levels of cortisol, an important hormone that helps regulate stress levels. Lower cortisol levels can increase the risk of PTSD.

In other words, the Holocaust victims' memories, experiences, and traumas influenced gene expression in their descendants. This could be applied to other traumas, including the transatlantic slave trade, inquisition, or war on terror. (4)

According to Ancestry.com, my DNA consists of forty-nine percent (49%) Ashkenazi Jew. As far back as I have been able to research, circa 1830, my father's family were Ashkenazi Jews from the Ukraine. I have never uncovered family members who were directly impacted by the Holocaust, but I did uncover an interesting genetic connection.

Israeli and American researchers investigating a healthy Ashkenazi Jewish population have identified a new genetic risk factor for schizophrenia and bipolar disorder (manic-depression)." Their work, just published in Nature Communications (2013), was reported by scientists at the Feinstein Institute for Medical Research in Manhasset, New York, and at the Hebrew University of Jerusalem.

The researchers identified the defect in the NDST3 gene by studying more than 25,000 individuals. (5)

Recent studies have suggested that neurological diseases can also be caused by epigenetic anomalies.

As interesting as all this emerging science or theory is, it doesn't answer my questions. Did all my family members suffer from diseases of similar DNA mutations? Perhaps with some epigenetics thrown in for good luck? Will future generations share the same fate?

I do know that being of Ashkenazi descent, I have a higher incidence of breast cancer. When I was diagnosed with breast cancer in 2022, I was tested for the BRCA gene mutation. Everyone carries this gene, but an inherited gene mutation is rare in the general population. In the United States, it is about one in 400 people, but among Ashkenazi Jewish men and women, about one in forty have a BRCA1/2 mutation. (6) I did not have it. And with three daughters and two granddaughters, I was happy to pass on these results.

I am a genealogist. I jumped on the DNA bandwagon quite early. With the advent of the Human Genome Project that technically began in 1990 (but actually earlier), the possibilities seemed endless. It planned to systematically map the entire human genome by the year 2005. It was announced in April 2003 that the project was completed, and the Human Genome Project gave us the ability to read nature's complete genetic blueprint for a human.

In a June 2000 White House event, President Bill Clinton announced,

Today, we are learning the language in which God created life. We are gaining ever more awe for the complexity, the beauty, the wonder of God's most divine and sacred gift. With this profound new knowledge, humankind is on the verge of gaining immense new power to heal. Genome science will have a real impact on all our lives—and even more, on the lives of our children.

It will revolutionize the diagnosis, prevention, and treatment of most, if not all, human diseases.

He concluded that the decoding of the genome was key to the greatest age of discovery ever known. (7)

Of course, the ethical and social questions remain and are numerous.

PART 6 – COPING

The Stigma

The stigma of mental illness has been around for millennia. In fact, in ancient Greece, a stigma was a brand to mark slaves or criminals. Those suffering from depression, schizophrenia, bipolar disorder, and other mental illnesses were not treated much better. They were imprisoned, tortured, or killed. During the Middle Ages, mental illness was regarded as a punishment from God.

Arthur Miller, the famous playwright, had a son with Down syndrome. I can't hear the name Arthur Miller without thinking of his most famous work, *Death of a Salesman*, which also brings to mind my father, 'The Peddler.' In *Death of a Salesman*, Willy Loman suffers from a mental illness, some say he was bipolar, like Dad. Miller and his wife kept the existence of their son a secret. They institutionalized him, as they were encouraged to do by doctors embracing the practice of the day regarding mental illness. The institution was close enough to home that Miller's wife would visit her son, but Miller never did.

There has long been a misconception that mental illnesses happen to people with flawed characters or moral failures of some kind, but it can happen to anyone.

Thankfully, the stigma of mental illness has evolved since the Middle Ages and even Arthur Miller's time. Along with medical, genetic, and biogenetic research, the dawn of social media has helped in many ways, allowing people to find resources as well as others with the same disorders. Of course, now we also have to deal with the negative side, the bullying, etc. But the world has opened wide enough for those suffering to see they are not alone.

Biogenetic explanations are reducing the blame that is attached to having a mental illness. *I am not alone—* and—*it's not my fault.* The lower the stigma, the more open the communication can become.

Many celebrities are openly talking about their mental illnesses.

Carrie Fisher, famously known as Princess Leia, was diagnosed as bipolar in her early twenties. She frequently talked about and wrote about her issues.

One of the things that baffles me (and there are quite a few) is how there can be so much lingering stigma with regards to mental illness, specifically bipolar disorder. In my opinion, living with manic depression takes a tremendous amount of balls. Not unlike a tour of Afghanistan (though the bombs and bullets, in this case, come from the inside). At times, being bipolar can be an all-consuming challenge, requiring a lot of stamina and even more courage, so if you're living with this illness and functioning at all, it's something to be proud of, not ashamed of.

They should issue medals along with the steady stream of medication.

~ Carrie Fisher (*Wishful Drinking*, 2008)

Singer Demi Lovato was diagnosed with bipolar disorder at age 22.

She chose to use her fame to help eliminate the stigma of mental illness. She took part in a campaign called Be Vocal: Speak Up for Mental Health in 2015.

Lovato said she wants women to know that "it's possible to live well, feel well, and also find happiness with bipolar disorder or any other mental illness they're struggling with."

Advocacy by people like these in the spotlight of our society continues to help dispel the stigma of mental illness discrimination, promote treatment, and give people hope.

Actress Glenn Close founded Bring Change 2 Mind, a nonprofit group dedicated to eliminating the stigma of mental illness. Her sister Jess had suffered from undiagnosed bipolar disorder for most of her life. Close confided:

We didn't talk about this ... we were a family with absolutely no vocabulary for mental illness, so Jess wasn't diagnosed until her late forties. Actually, her son was diagnosed before she was.

Give families the words they need to overcome fear about mental illness and start talking.

What mental health needs is more sunlight, more candor, and more unashamed conversation. (6)

She uses the hashtag #EndtheStigma.

Stigma is not just what other people think, but it translates into keeping the mentally ill from seeking care for themselves. Often, people avoid seeking help because they are worried about being treated differently or labeled or fear losing their jobs or relationships. It also translates into our shortage of mental health professionals, access to care, and a lack of investments in enough resources for the mentally ill.

We've Come a Long Way

Treatments for all types of mental illness have come a long way since the 1950s and 1960s. Thousands of years ago and even as recently as the eighteenth and nineteenth centuries, a mentally ill person was considered possessed with evil spirits or accused of witchcraft.

The treatments? There was a time when witches were burned. Other treatments included: trephination—a surgical intervention in which a hole is drilled into the human skull, bloodletting, lobotomy—which involves severing connections in the brain's prefrontal cortex, isolation, commitment to asylums, and sterilization.

Electroconvulsive (electroshock) therapy is still used today but has vastly improved from the days when my father and my sister received them. According to the National Institutes of Health, there have been many changes since the 1930s in:

1. Pulse width

2. Dosing and duration

3. Electrode placement

4. Safety concerns

5. Using anesthesia, muscle relaxants

The current practice today is known as modified electroconvulsive therapy (ECT). In the early years, there was no use of anesthesia or muscle relaxants, which often would cause seizures, pain, or even broken bones. Today, ECT is performed by delivering an electrical current to a patient's brain via electrodes placed on the scalp to induce a seizure while the patient is under anesthesia and a muscle relaxant. ECT's exact mechanism of action is unknown, but researchers believe it may relieve depressive symptoms by regulating functional disturbances in relevant neural circuits. (1)

As far as schizophrenic treatments are concerned, it became apparent that both insulin coma and leucotomy (similar to lobotomy) were ineffective and could cause serious side effects, even proving fatal. Deep insulin coma therapy (DICT) was the treatment for schizophrenia from the late 1930s until the late 1950s when the first antipsychotic chlorpromazine (Thorazine) came into use. It was also eventually discovered that ECT was ineffective in schizophrenia.

Regarding sterilization, the infamous 1927 Supreme Court Case Buck v. Bell (2) upheld a State of Virginia statute permitting the sterilization of the "so-called intellectually unfit." "Three generations of imbeciles are enough," was the famous quote from Supreme Court Judge Oliver Wendell Holmes.

Carrie Buck was a feeble-minded white woman committed to a state institution. She was the daughter of a feeble-minded mother in the same institution and the mother of an illegitimate feeble-minded child. She was eighteen years old at the time of the trial in circuit court in 1924. The case was lost at the Supreme Court, and Carrie Buck was sterilized.

As we moved into the twentieth century, it was generally accepted that biological and environmental factors caused mental illness. However, it was well into the mid-twentieth century when such procedures as lobotomies were finally stopped as a treatment. The last recorded lobotomy in the United States was performed by Dr. Walter Freeman in 1967 and ended in the death of the patient.

Today, this treatment is obsolete. It did, however, win a Nobel Prize in Physiology and Medicine in 1949. Popular in the 1940s and 1950s, lobotomies were always controversial and were only prescribed in psychiatric cases thought to be most severe.

Rosemary Kennedy, the sister of John F and Robert Kennedy, had a lobotomy in 1941.

For many years, the American public knew little about the eldest Kennedy daughter, Rosemary. Her life inspired her family members to take up work for people with intellectual and physical disabilities.

In their search for cures for Rosemary, the Kennedys learned about a new experimental procedure, a lobotomy. This brain surgery would supposedly reduce depression and aggressiveness in patients but was not yet accepted by the American Medical Association. While there were many examples of failed cases, those pioneering the surgery assured Joe Kennedy of its promise of success. In November 1941, Mr. Kennedy arranged to have a lobotomy performed on Rosemary. It was immediately clear that the operation had drastically failed. Rosemary had lost most of her ability to walk or talk. Her personality had been forever altered, and she was left physically disabled. After being released from the hospital, Rosemary was immediately institutionalized. (3)

She remained institutionalized for the rest of her life.

The more I learn about the Kennedys, the more grateful I am for their activism in the field of mental illness. I imagine because of what happened to their sister Rosemary, they took up the mantle, took advantage of their high-profile lives, and advocated for the mentally ill.

I am also aware of the personal connection I have from their moving to Riverdale in the late 1920s, before I was born, to when Bobby (Robert F.) Kennedy, then a U.S. Senator from New York, had paid an unannounced visit to Willowbrook in 1965 and denounced its conditions calling it a "snake pit" with residents living "in filth and dirt ... in rooms less comfortable and cheerful than the cages for animals in a zoo."

Then there was the president, John F. Kennedy, who made mental illness and disabilities a priority of his new administration. He established the National Institute of Child Health and Human Development. In 1963, he signed the Maternal and Child Health and Mental Retardation Planning Amendment to the Social Security Act, the first major legislation to combat mental illness and intellectual disabilities.

Eunice (Kennedy) Shriver, sister to Robert and John, was a great catalyst to her politician brothers. She was always a great advocate and friend to Rosemary. She worked for people with intellectual disabilities her entire life. She and Rosemary would always play sports together growing up and, in 1962, she had the idea of inviting young people with intellectual disabilities to a summer camp she hosted in her backyard. She called it Camp Shriver.

Today, what started as Camp Shriver in Eunice's backyard is now the Special Olympics. Today, more than six million children and adults in more than two hundred countries participate in the Special Olympics.

It is a relief that twenty-first-century attitudes around mental illness are more open, accepting, and sympathetic. We still have a long way to go, but this has led to more sharing of painful and troubling issues surrounding matters of the mind. The World Health Organization's guidelines state that promoting mental health is integral to public health. WHO stresses that mental health is more than the absence of mental illness; there is no health without mental health.

John F. Kennedy passed the Community Mental Health Act of 1963. It established a system of community-based care instead of institutional care for people with mental illness like my brother Warren, and no doubt was instrumental in closing down institutions like Willowbrook School. In 2023, It was announced that the current administration would award nearly $130 Million to expand certified community behavioral health clinics across the US. This continues to deliver on the promise of the 1963 Act by strengthening the care available in the community.

Hope for Genetic Research

According to the National Institute of Mental Health:

One day, genetic research may make it possible to provide a more complete picture of a person's risk of getting a particular mental disorder or to diagnose it based on his or her genes. Although recent studies have begun to identify the genetic markers associated with certain mental disorders and eventually may lead to better screening and more personalized treatment, it is still too early to use genetic tests or genome scans to diagnose or treat mental disorders accurately. For example, the Genomics Research Branch of the NIMH is currently studying and supporting research on the human genetic variations that contribute to the risk for mood and anxiety disorders, such as bipolar disorder and panic disorder, so that better ways to diagnose and treat these disorders can be developed. (1)

Cancer used to be a death sentence, and not all that long ago. Just like we can live a good life and thrive after cancer, so it is with mental illnesses. The old lines 'pull yourself together' and 'everything will be alright' no longer hold much water. How we see and treat mental illness in the twenty-first century has changed. Instead of asylums and "snake pit" institutions, there are psychiatric hospitals emphasizing short-term stays, an abundance of drugs available, virtual therapy, and telemedicine, which is especially valuable in rural areas, where access to mental health specialists is limited. Research has found that teletherapy is as effective as in-person treatment in most cases.

It is more usual these days that people consult psychologists, psychiatrists, therapists, counselors, clinical social workers, and religious leaders. This, too, is because of lessening the stigma of mental illness.

Psychiatric genetics has made substantial progress in the last decade, providing new insights into the genetic etiology of psychiatric disorders and paving the way for precision psychiatry, in which individual genetic profiles may be used to personalize risk assessment and inform clinical decision-making.

Pharmacogenomics deals precisely with this issue area. It is defined as the study of variability in drug response due to the genetic code. Genetic screening in clinical practice will hopefully become routine soon, enabling psychiatrists to customize drug treatment to achieve better efficacy and tolerability for each patient. This will help us adapt therapies to address genetic variations within our ethnically diverse society.

Hope for Schizophrenia Treatment

One of the most critical advances in the treatment of schizophrenia has been the discovery of antipsychotic drugs like chlorpromazine that reduce the symptoms. It ushered in a new era of treatment for psychiatric illness and gave people the chance to live normal lives.

The first large-scale clinical trials of chlorpromazine and other antipsychotic drugs were conducted in the United States in the early 1960s. Since then, over two hundred clinical trials of antipsychotics in schizophrenia have been published. Taken together, they show that antipsychotics lead to a greater improvement in the symptoms of schizophrenia.

Although current antipsychotics are far from perfect, as they can cause a wide range of side effects and not all people respond to them, the existence of a range of antipsychotics reduces these problems to a degree, as people who find that one drug doesn't suit them have the option of switching to another. Nevertheless, it is clear that new and better treatments for schizophrenia and psychosis are needed so that more people with these disorders can recover and lead active lives, and also so that there is a greater choice of treatment.

Joshua Kantrowitz, associate professor of clinical psychiatry at Columbia University, said,

For a long time, we've really only been treating some of the symptoms of schizophrenia and treating them indirectly, but having new treatments that work in different ways will make it possible to start fine-tuning

which symptoms respond to which drug and why. We're still not really addressing the root cause of the disease, but perhaps, slowly but surely, we'll get there. (1)

Hope for Technological Advances

Article courtesy of University of Texas Southwestern Medical Center Newsroom:

Artificial intelligence may soon play a critical role in choosing which depression therapy is best for patients.

A national trial initiated by University of Texas Southwestern in 2011 to better understand mood disorders has produced what scientists are calling the project's flagship finding: a computer that can accurately predict whether an antidepressant will work based on a patient's brain activity.

The new research is the latest among several studies from the trial that cumulatively show how high-tech strategies can help doctors objectively diagnose and prescribe depression treatments. Although implementing these approaches will take time, researchers predict tools such as AI, brain imaging, and blood tests will revolutionize the field of psychiatry in the coming years.

The future of psychiatry will likely be increasingly personalized. Over time, technology will play a more significant role in how mental health conditions are detected, diagnosed, and treated. (1)

I have read articles that say AI could be a more useful tool than a psychotherapy session with a human doctor. A growing body of evidence suggests that AI can help diagnose conditions, develop therapies, and enable more personalized approaches and treatments.

On the other hand, just as many articles and studies refute this fact. There, of course, are the ethical issues—concerns about bias, fairness, equity, justice, and privacy. AI in medicine also raises significant legal and ethical challenges. Several of these concerns are about privacy, discrimination, psychological harm, and the physician-patient relationship. How much empathy and sympathy can artificial intelligence emote? I can't help picturing a distraught patient being hugged by a robot.

One example is Woebot. A therapeutic chatbot (2) is a chatbot that learns to adapt to its users' personalities and is capable of talking them through a number of therapies and talking exercises commonly used to help patients learn to cope with various conditions. Woebot's website comes with this caveat:

Woebot for Adults is a non-prescription medical device under FDA enforcement discretion; it is not evaluated, cleared, or approved by FDA. It is not a prescription product. It is not intended to diagnose, monitor, treat, or prevent any disease. It may be considered an adjunct to clinical care but does not replace clinical care.

Another chatbot, Tess (3), offers free 24/7 on-demand emotional support and can be used to help cope with anxiety and panic attacks whenever they occur. The website shows a very simple three-step process:

1. Enter your phone number, and Tess will text you.

2. Tess will ask, "How are you?" You reply by telling Tess what's bothering you.

3. Tess makes you feel better by chatting with you.

Though I can see where this could be beneficial in some cases, especially in rural areas or where people have no one to confide in or are just plain afraid to reveal what they are going through, in the event of trying to assess such things as suicide risk, there would have to be some very close coordination between the bot and the healthcare worker.

According to the Medical Futurist,

AI can give a helping hand when it comes to the early detection of depression. The machine learning algorithm created at Vanderbilt University Medical Center in Nashville uses hospital admissions data, including age, gender, zip code, medication, and diagnostic history, to predict the likelihood of any given individual taking their own life. In trials using data gathered from more than 5,000 patients who had been admitted to the hospital for either self-harm or suicide attempts, the algorithm was 84 percent accurate at predicting whether someone would attempt suicide the following week and 80 percent accurate at predicting whether someone would attempt suicide within the following two years. (4)

AI can also detect depression from your voice—and it's even eerily accurate. In fact, it's twice as accurate in it than a human.

A recent Pew Research Center survey indicated that sixty percent of Americans would be uncomfortable with provider relying on AI in their own healthcare. (1) Of course, that may decrease as we get used to AI, especially if it is a successful practitioner.

"There might be as many as 1,000 smartphone-based 'biomarkers' for depression," said Dr. Thomas Insel, former head of the National Institute of Mental Health and now a leader in the smartphone psychiatry movement. Researchers are testing apps that use artificial intelligence to try to predict depression episodes or potential self-harm.

The smartphone psychiatry movement! That's a new one.

According to an article in The Atlantic by David Dobbs, Tom Insel is now trying to reduce the world's anguish through the devices in people's pockets:

Smartphones can track daily behaviors that reflect mental health. A phone can sense the beginning of a crisis and trigger an appropriate treatment response. (5)

There are also Facebook-like apps for groups, say, who have all had a psychotic episode or a suicide attempt and connect them with each other and health professionals who are available on these apps. Of course, like any other social media application, it could be a prime target for exploitation. Whether or not this is the future of psychiatry and treating mental illness, I don't know. But I do find it fascinating. I wonder what those practitioners of the eighteenth century would have thought.

Hope for Mental Health Parity

One great stride of the twenty-first century is the passage of federal laws to equalize coverage between mental health and physical health. The Mental Health Parity and Addiction Equity Act of 2008 (MHPAEA or Parity Law) "requires most health plans or health insurers that offer coverage for mental health conditions or substance use disorders to make these benefits comparable to those offered for medical and surgical benefits."(1) And the Affordable Care Act (ACA) of 2010 extended the Mental Health Parity and Addiction Equity Act (MHPAEA) to individual and small group plans. Even though these acts have been passed, that doesn't mean they have fully been enforced. Compliance with mental health parity means working to ensure that when a person seeks treatment for a mental health condition or substance use disorder under the health coverage that they were promised through their employment, that treatment is available just as easily as it is for any medical condition. There is an immense amount of work left to do.

The development of new treatments and the gradual decrease in stigma about seeking help are providing optimism for the future.

PART 7 - TRACES

Legacy

A few years ago, my mother got to that stage of life where she told my sisters and me that she would rather die on the bathroom floor at home (which is where she had recently been found) than stay where she was in the nursing home. I had just read a book that my sister Stacey recommended on the subject of closing the communication gap with our elders called, *How to Say it to Seniors,* by David Solie. (1) It was pretty simple in its premise.

Basically, what we all are looking for in our elderly years is:

• Maintain control
• A legacy

Well, Mom was maintaining control, refusing the long-term care and doing it her way.

But what about the legacy?

Mom was always a writer, mostly poetry and children's stories. Growing up, I remember that she was constantly sending large manila envelopes out in the mail. Her cute, upbeat poems were frequently published in our hometown newspaper. She was very proud of that fact, and I realized that the older she got, she constantly talked about her writing (even though she hadn't written anything in probably forty years).

In David Solie's book, he explained these phenomena as 'searching for a legacy'" We all have experienced older people constantly talking about their past accomplishments. Sometimes, there are stories we never heard before. They are trying to find the things in their lives that they want to be remembered by—their legacy.

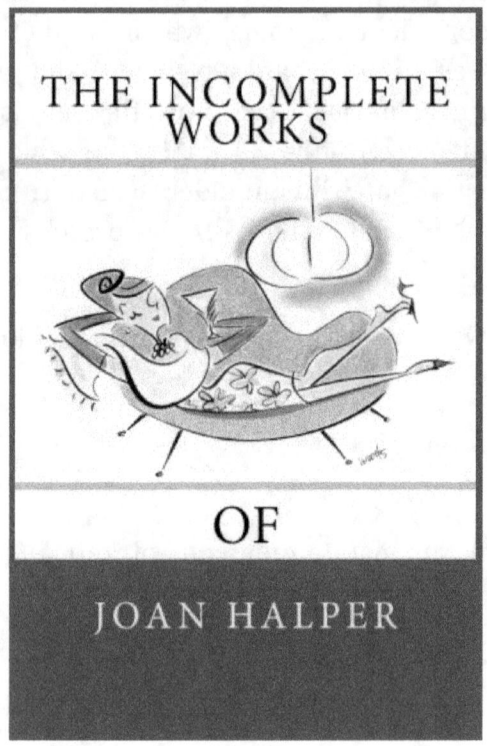

Cover art by Sharon Watts

I believed that my mother wanted her legacy to be that of a writer. Unbeknownst to my mother, I collected all the writings I could find and self-published a little book on Amazon called *The Incomplete Works of Joan Halper*. It was incomplete because she was still alive at the time and always said she wanted to write again. Unfortunately, she had macular degeneration and could hardly see.

When publishing was complete, I sent a box of twenty-five books to my sister's house.

Mom didn't see very well, so I wasn't sure she would understand what they were. Plus, I figured she would want to share the moment.

Well, she was absolutely floored. She told me that no one in her life had ever done something as wonderful as this for her. She autographed each one, gave them to friends, and gave them to her doctors. I'm surprised she has not yet given one to a stranger. She told me people had even started "treating her differently" since she published a book. I've said to her, "You are telling them that it's self-published, right?" She said yes ... but I doubt it.

Which brings me to this *mishegoss* of a book here, keeping the legacy of my family alive. It was a family full of complicated people and complicated issues. A family full of people who did not get to live their best lives or even a very long life. But they lived the best they could with what they were dealt. And those of us who survived are dealing with the aftermath as best we can. I think for most of us, there has been forgiveness and understanding.

Lorraine: She has been gone for fifty-six years in October 2023. She has a legacy. She was a sister, a daughter, a friend. She was a semifinalist in a beauty pageant and wrote poetry. She had friends and family who loved her in her seventeen short years.

Warren, the 'not forgotten': To be brutally honest, he was forgotten by our family for many, many years. Reasons and excuses aside, I hope to bring him to life on these pages and tell his story. To see him in person after fifty years has been such a thrill.

Burt (Dad): Probably the most complicated of all. I've related stories funny and horrific, and there's not much more I can say. I know that he hoped his writings, *Pieces of My Mind*, would be his legacy.

Perhaps I became a genealogist so my children and grandchildren would have a more expanded legacy than the story I have just told. Brave ancestors crossed the ocean, not knowing what was on the other side. Ancestors fought in wars from the Revolutionary War to World War II. The battles were physical as well as mental.

Your ancestors are the individuals from whom you are biologically descended and connect genetics and society in fundamental ways.

The Agony and the Ecstasy

by Burton Halper

Excerpted from *Pieces of My Mind*, published in Veterans Administration Magazine

It is a mixed blessing to be a manic-depressive. In my manic state, with the total absence of fear, I felt as if I were on a mountainous peak of infallibility, and then conversely was the unbearable pain of depression, which left me in an emotional straitjacket incapable of doing even the simplest of tasks. It gave me feelings of hopelessness and fear. And then again, not too long afterward, I would be rocketed into an ecstatic high. It was as if I was suddenly transformed from a fearful, vulnerable, puny excuse for a man to a superman.

My manic state gave me a newly found self-confidence, which was responsible for my success as a salesman. I sold to virtually everyone, whether they wanted or needed my product. I mesmerized them with my contagious enthusiasm, and the power and control I had acquired gave me the feeling of invincibility.

My ESP was uncanny because, with the process of thought and visualization, I was thrown into the right place at the right time.

I can remember when it was virtually impossible to find a parking place, and then one would suddenly appear just through positive thought. I now grieve for the euphoric times, but with the knowledge that would come from the stabilizing effect of the drug lithium, the price to be paid

by the pain of depression would be too costly a price to be paid.

Without the fear of failure, painting a picture in oils was no longer intimidating. I not only got a great deal of joy, but I also experienced euphoria upon its completion, which rivaled a sexual one. I needed the reassurance that the painting I created was not just an illusion, and when all my friends wanted copies of my painting, that was all the reassurance I needed. They were real, and they were good, and I created them.

Another creative interest I have would probably never have surfaced if not for my manic depressive disease. My mania inspired me to write over one hundred fifty autobiographical short stories, which I call the collection A Piece of My Mind. Many of the stories were published in the National Veteran's Voice magazine, and I know that they were well written because of the acclaim I received from a doctor of literature at the University of New Mexico.

My bipolar disorder has been truly a double-edged sword. I could never have had the pleasure from the high manic states if I didn't have the pain of being depressed. I feel blessed for the suffering I had to endure so that I could experience the heights of euphoria. I grieve over the loss of my mania.

Life and Death

by Burton Halper

Not to be able to finish all the things undone—the unfinished painting, book, the unresolved petty arguments and grievances, the interrupted vicarious wealth that could have become reality.

If given just a little more time. The recognition, acceptance, and respect so much needed, the marriage and future happiness of his children, never being referred to as Grandpa or bouncing them on his knee, or tucking them in.

The unresolved, unfinished differences with a wife, mother, sweetheart, friend who was always there to fill the void of loneliness and despair, and the receptacle of mutual pleasure manifesting itself into six unique personalities that may give me a semblance of immortality.

Never will the fantasy of a beautiful, sensual, voluptuous mistress be fulfilled, having an insatiable longing to love and be loved.

With all the unfinished, unseen, and unfulfilled vicarious thoughts, he has been truly blessed that his life was never a mere existence. It has been lived to the fullest in his deepest despair or highest euphoria.

His legacy, although not tangible, lies in the intrinsic value through his philosophy and writings; the priceless knowledge of living life to its fullest.

Of his six offspring, I am the only child to make him a Grandpa, so he did get to 'bounce them on his knee.' I'm happy about that. Dad passed away in 1999, at the age of sixty-nine, from heart failure.

Kind Heaven

by Lorraine Halper

How gentle is the rain
falling on moistened eyes
stained with tears washing
away what caused
the expression of sadness.
Heaven's kind water

How gentle is the sun
warm upon my face
bright to shield me from
darkness.
Heaven's sweet rays of light

How gentle is the wind
whispering words of coolness
and tranquility
A soothing breeze easing
all discomfort

A stronger wind now blowing warning
me of changing times unsteadiness
and fear arise.
The gentle rain now ice hard
and cold—dreariness

The sun, no longer warm
no longer bright.
Darkness falls upon me

Where is the gentle rain to
wash away my tears the
warm bright sun upon my
face to shield me from
darkness?
The gentle wind whispering

words of coolness and tranquility?

Gone, all is gone and passing. Where
is what was once
so beautiful, so peaceful?

Have faith, the rain cries
The sun impresses
The wind whispers.
Strive for another change it
will come and in
Greater quantity.

Lorraine wrote poetry, too. I found this to be quite profound. It is not dated, so I have no idea how close this writing was to her suicide. Did the change ever come before it left for good? Could any of us been able to be part of that change?

Imagine

by Marlene Dunham

I strive but fail
to imagine how it would feel
if I were to be a
firefly, a butterfly,
free from a human kind
of soul or the mind of that
sister, father, brother, friend
that could not open the door
to reality
so sadly,
made other plans.

I imagine what it would be like
to have no control or desire,

for that matter, to live a life of
any kind; to find a reason even to
open your eyes each day.
To face life's constant strains

I imagine standing on the edge of
that ledge looking at the street
below bottomless, ultimate,
critical the pivotal point where
sanity's drowned and all else
becomes irrelevant

Those thoughts hold firm
and won't unhinge its grasp.
Convinced that
peace will be at the
canyon's floor

I can't imagine...

I mourn for the psyche

of those beautiful minds;
while I celebrate the
simple fact
that
I, can't imagine.

My own reply to all of these family members with mental illness who I have written about (my sister, my father, and my brother), is that I cannot imagine what they had to go through. I still ask, "Why not me?" And even though I can't imagine what it was like, and for that, I am thankful. I am more confident now that my children and grandchildren will not have to endure what members of my family had to. And with the advances in science, gene therapies, DNA, pharmacology, etc., many future generations may not either.

I never want them forgotten, however, nor the plight of the mentally ill. I am thankful for all the public, political, and medical advances that have happened these past decades and the continuation of advocacy, research, and just plain caring about our fellow human beings.

Imagine all the people
living for today.

~ John Lennon

IN CONCLUSION

I feel guilty when I say that I always thought of myself as relatively normal, although my ex-husband would probably not agree. Maybe even my children would disagree with me on that at times in my life. As my brother Bruce has said, it's like a bolt of lightning struck our family, but not every member. I am very grateful that the hereditary DNA of bipolar 1, schizophrenia, or level 3 autism was never passed down to me, my children, or my grandchildren.

I've divulged a little about promiscuity in my early twenties, drug use in the early seventies, and the fifteen years I spent in a fundamentalist religious cult. It could be construed that it was because I didn't have enough love and attention, like Claudia says. Or that I never had a father figure, so I looked to the 'man of God' for that. I suppose that transgenerational epigenetics from all the trauma I grew up around could have been an influence on how I lived my life, but that, my friends, is for another book.

As you focus on clearing your generational trauma,
do not forget to claim your
generational strengths.
Your ancestors gave you more than just wounds.

~ Anonymous

EPILOGUE: The Reunion with Warren

October 10, 2023 – Turner Road, Plattsburgh, New York

The letter from his caseworker said,

The plan will be for us to go to Warren's home and have coffee with him, which he does every day at 2pm. Then we can visit with him in his favorite spot, the screened in porch! He loves to be out there so it will allow him to be comfortable and give you two privacy to catch up! I can't guarantee a quiet visit, I am not sure of what the plans are for Warren's housemates during this time, but the porch will allow a quiet visit as I feel that the porch is Warren's Man Cave, and no one usually goes out there but Warren. He has his favorite chair and favorite weighted blanket out there for his comfort.

It had been fifty years for me. The last time I saw Warren was soon after he had been moved to Willowbrook. I don't remember going more than once, as it was such a creepy place. I was twenty years old, off to college and off to the rest of my life. Not long after, I moved from New York to Washington State and the rest of the family moved on to Arizona. I often wondered if part of their decision was to feel less guilty about not visiting Warren at Willowbrook.

For years, Stacey didn't know she had another living brother, just like she didn't know she had a sister who had passed away. Stacey had never met Warren. He was institutionalized eight years before she was even born and apparently, there were no pictures of him hanging on the walls of our apartment.

The plan was hatched. October 2023 seemed the best time for the trip. I told Stacey I would love her to come with me and meet her brother for the first time. She was a bit reluctant at first, a bit anxious, but plans were made and we met up in Montreal. She flew from San Francisco and I flew from Seattle. Warren resided in Plattsburgh, New York, which was only about a sixty-three-mile drive from Montreal. No disrespect to Plattsburgh, but we thought it would be much more fun to stay in Montreal for three or four days. My sister came armed with the names of all the foodie places we had seen on the TV show Somebody Feed Phil. Phil Rosenthal, better known as the creator of Everybody Loves Raymond, travels to different cities throughout the world and highlights their food and culture. One of those cities was Montreal. I'm not sure what was more popular, the show or the chicken restaurant we tried the first night, *Ma Poule Mouillee*. Translation: The Wet Chicken. Despite the name, it was obviously very popular. There was a line about two blocks long, that of course, we stood in. About forty minutes later, with chicken and poutine in hand, we went back to our Airbnb to eat it. Not bad – and not really 'wet.'

After spending two days in the rain and traffic of Quebec, we were ready for our drive south. Montreal was very nice, aside from the traffic and road construction and a detour every other block. Unfortunately, Hertz thought they were doing me a favor when they gave me a free upgrade to a Chrysler 300. My advice: Don't try to drive a Chrysler 300 down Rue St. Paul. But we really did enjoy Montreal.

We had arranged to meet both Warren's care manager and his advocate from the New York State Office for People with Developmental Disabilities (OPWDD) for lunch in a nearby café.

OPWDD was created in 1978 as an independent cabinet-level state agency, largely because of the need for an autonomous entity to implement the Willowbrook consent decree and the resulting closure and downsizing of Willowbrook and other large institutions. In the decades that followed, it has become one of the state's largest agencies.

I was heartened to learn of the care that the State of New York is giving to those with developmental disabilities and the extra care for the Willowbrook Class. Meeting these two women in that café was proof enough of the care and concern that my brother is getting. They spent two hours with my sister and me talking about Warren, listening to us recount our own family history, and answering any questions that they were able. They could not have been more caring and sincere. I am so grateful to have met them.

Not only did they spend those two hours talking with us but also went with us to meet Warren. He was familiar with both of them, so they carved out even more of their very busy days to come along.

We arrived at the house on Turner Road. It was out in the country among the trees. The feeling was peaceful and bucolic. His house manager greeted us and let us know that the other housemates had gone out so that we would have more privacy and less chaos.

There are four male house members. I believe at age sixty-eight, Warren is the oldest. Two of the men are more high functioning and a bit outspoken, while Warren is essentially mute and very low functioning. The fourth member falls somewhere in between and it all works.

The house manager told us that Warren had just gone to his room to lie down. His advocate went and peeked her head in his room to say "Warren, you have some company. Do you want to come out and say hello?" No response. His habit is to get into his bed with his legs crossed in a yoga position, then pull the blanket over his head and lie down. He looked like a not so little cocoon. I then said, "Hello Warren, I brought you a present" and

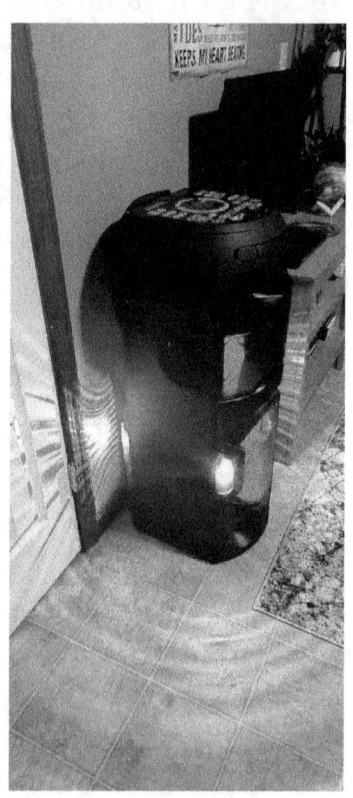

he immediately popped up from his bed and ran down the hall to the dining room table. He moves very quickly (and apparently even more quickly when there is a present involved).

For someone who becomes overstimulated very easily I was quite surprised to see his room. There were colored lights everywhere, even a disco ball hanging from the ceiling. He had the biggest, coolest radio, CD, and speaker combination I'd seen in a while. Music is everything to him. It calms him.

A bit later, we went out to his favorite spot on the porch where he sits in his lounge chair to rock and listen to music. We went through his box of vinyl albums sitting next to the record player. I was a bit surprised. I had to laugh and think, "He's a man after my own heart". There was Pink Floyd, Led Zeppelin, Fleetwood Mac, The Beatles (his favorite) and even AC/DC and Metallica!

So, Warren came out of his room to get his present. I brought him a Seattle Sweatshirt, as I know he loves sweatshirts. He went straight to the kitchen to get strawberry milk. The house manager poured his milk and then let him pour in the strawberry syrup and mix it up. They brought it to the table where he gulped it down as fast as he could and some of it landed down the front of his shirt. Apparently, all those years at Willowbrook ingrained in him that everyone would steal his food if they could, so eating it or drinking it as fast as he could was the only way to protect it. To this day, he has to have someone watch him eat so the food doesn't go down too fast and choke him. When a new member of the household is added, Warren will either bring his food to his room or else put his arm around the plate, protecting it from the would-be food thief. Once he is comfortable with the new house member, he will come back to the table for meals. It has been thirty-eight years since Warren left Willowbrook. Habits die hard. It is very difficult to change a long-standing pattern of behavior. I only wish I knew what other horrible memories reside in his brain from spending his most formative years at Willowbrook State School.

He came to the dining room table and sat across from me. We looked at each other. There was a connection of some sort. I asked if it was alright to take a picture. His advocate asked Warren if it would be okay and he immediately jumped up from the table. I thought, "Oh no, he's going to run back to his room, and turn back into a cocoon." To my surprise, however, he stood up, went to the middle of the room and looked right at me, as if to say, "I'm ready for my picture now." I thought I would quickly take advantage of the situation and handed my phone to Stacey and asked her to take a picture of both of us. I nonchalantly went over and stood next to Warren.

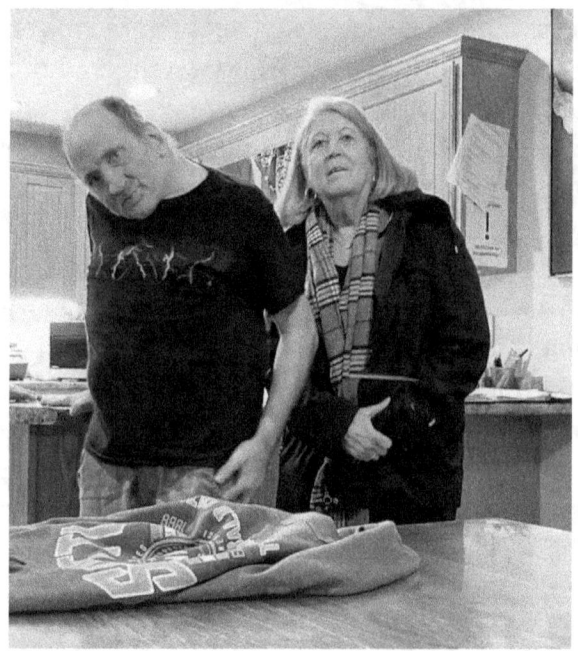

Warren has scoliosis, which is why his head is bent to the right. Other than that, for a sixty-eight-year-old man, he is pretty good health – considering what he has been through. I am sure the question of why he has no fingertips will never be answered.

At one point Warren grabbed my arm and started pulling me towards the kitchen. I thought this was a real moment between us, but it turned out he wanted more strawberry milk. When I realized, I just laughed and said, "Oh, he's just using me."

We probably had a total of twenty minutes or so until Warren decided to go back to his room, get in his bed, and pull the blanket back over his head. Stacey, for the most part, stayed in the background. But I know she was as moved as I was by the whole experience.

I wanted him to touch my ears. He reached out and touched my hand once. And I really believe we did have a connection, my brother and I.

His caseworker emailed me after I got home, "I felt that Warren made a special connection with you, Marlene, the way he looked at you as if to say, 'I know who that is, but I can't place the where or the why I know her.'"

From the chapter, After Willowbrook in Part 3, I wrote,

I only pray that when I go for my first visit in fifty years, he will have a sense of who I am, a recognition that we belong together somehow, like pieces of the puzzle that was once our family.

Lastly, the synchronicity of it all:

The date we went to see Warren (October 10th) was the 56th anniversary of the death of Lorraine. October 10, 1967.

MARLENE DUNHAM

Endnotes and References

Part 1 – The Family Begins. Birth Control

Endnote (1) Noonan, J. T. Contraception: A History of Its Treatment by the Catholic Theologians and Canonists, Enlarged Edition (Harvard University Press, 2012

Part 2 – Family Secrets. Another Reality

Reference:
http://www.mayoclinic.com/health/electroconvulsive-therapy/MY00129

Robert Lowell Walking in the Blue - Public Domain Poetry. this poetry is now in the public domain, Robert Lowell (March 1, 1917 - September 12, 1977), born Robert Traill Spence Lowell, IV, was an American poet whose works, confessional in nature, engaged with the questions of history and probed the dark recesses of the self.

Part 2 – Family Secrets. Lithium

Endnote (1) Shorter, E. The History of Lithium Therapy. Bipolar Disorders, 11, 4-9.
https://onlinelibrary.wiley.com/doi/10.1111/j.1399-5618.2009.00706.x

Endnote (2)
https://en.wikipedia.org/wiki/Ronald_R._Fieve

References:

(3) Gershon S, Yuwiler A. Lithium-ion: A Specific Psychopharmacological Approach To The Treatment of Mania. J Neuropsychiatry. 1960;1:229–241.

Ruffalo ML. A Brief History https://pubmed.ncbi.nlm.nih.gov/29045768 2017

Lithium Manhattan Manic City by Ronald R Fieve, MD, Film: https://youtu.be/HLoGGa5NLHs

Part 3 - Institutions. Willowbrook

Endnote (1) https://en.wikipedia.org/wiki/Willowbrook_State_Sch ool

Endnote (2) Staff (September 10, 1965). "Excerpts From Statement by Kennedy." The New York Times. Retrieved September 26, 2010.

Endnote (3) Rivera, Geraldo (1972). Willowbrook: The Last Great Disgrace. WABC-TV. Archived from the original on 2014-03-02. Retrieved 2014-02-26

Endnote (4) University of Albany Library, Transcript of interview with Dr. William Bronston and Dr. Michael Wilkins, 2007 August 19. Accessed February 21, 2012. https://archives.albany.edu/downloads/6m311p28w?lo cale=en

Endnote (5) Consent Decree Rothman, D. J. and Rothman, S.M. (2005) The Willowbrook Wars: Bringing the Mentally Disabled into The Community. (New York, Transaction Publishers 2005

Endnote (6) Willowbrook Class

https://opwdd.ny.gov/system/files/documents/2019/11/willowbrook_permanent_injunction_lori_o.pdf

References:

Carabello, B.; Wilkins, Mike; Rivera, Geraldo; and College of Staten Island. Willowbrook the last disgrace—twenty-five years later. 2006, 1997. (Library Media Services. 2006).

Goode, D.; Hill, D.; and Reiss, J. History and Sociology of the Willowbrook State School. United States of America: (American Association on Intellectual and Developmental Disabilities 2013)

Data Research, Inc. (1994) Rehabilitation Act. Statutes, Regulations and Case Law Protecting Individuals with Disabilities

Rothman, D. J. and Rothman, S.M. (2005) The Willowbrook Wars: Bringing the Mentally Disabled Into the Community. (New York, Transaction Publishers 2005)

Part 3 - Institutions. After Willowbrook

References:

The Path Forward: Remembering Willowbrook: A conversation with Dr. Michael Wilkins and Bernard Carabello
https://www.youtube.com/watch?v=CM9fnwUp2iU
2023

National Council on Disability
https://ncd.gov/newsroom/05042015

College of Staten Island — The Willowbrook Mile
https://www.csi.cuny.edu/about-csi/president-
leadership/administration/office-vp-economic-
development-and-community-partnerships/reporting-
units-and-initiatives/willowbrook-mile/about

Part 4 – Different Perspectives. Lorraine

Endnote (1) https://www.nami.org/About-Mental-
Illness/Mental-Health-Conditions/Schizophrenia

Endnote (2) Koenig HG. Religion, Spirituality, and
Psychotic Disorders. Revista de Psiquiatria Clínica.
2007;34(1):40-48. doi:10.1590/S0101-
60832007000700013

Endnote (3) Szasz TS. The Myth of Mental Illness:
Foundations of a Theory of Personal Conduct. (Secker &
Warburg, 1962) https://www.amazon.com/Myth-
Mental-Illness-Foundations-Personal/dp/0061771228/

References:

Murray, ED.; Cunningham MG; "The Role of Psychotic
Disorders in Religious History Considered." (Price BH
2012)

Grover S, Davuluri T, Chakrabarti S. Religion,
Spirituality, and Schizophrenia: A Review. Indian J
Psychol Med. 2014;36(2):119-24. doi:10.4103/0253-
7176.130962

Part 4 – Different Perspectives, Bruce

Endnote (1) Steve Colbert quote
https://www.gq.com/story/stephen-colbert-gq-cover-story?

Part 5 – The DNA Connection, Autism

Endnote (1) https://www.verywellhealth.com/what-is-severe-autism-260044

References:
https://blogs.uoregon.edu/autismhistoryproject

Part 5 – The DNA Connection, Bipolar Disorder and Schizophrenia

Endnote (2)
https://www.medicalnewstoday.com/articles/324440

Endnote (3) Lithium, Its Role in Psychiatric Research and Treatment, edited by: Samuel Gershon and Baron Shopsin (New York: Plenum Press, 1973).

Part 5 – The DNA Connection, The Overlap

Endnote (1) Carroll, L.S., Owen, M.J. Genetic overlap between autism, schizophrenia and bipolar disorder. Genome Med 1, 102 (2009).
https://doi.org/10.1186/gm102

Endnote (2) Craddock N, O'Donovan MC, Owen MJ. The genetics of schizophrenia and bipolar disorder: dissecting psychosis. J Med Genet. 2005; 42:193–204. doi: 10.1136/jmg.2005.030718.

Endnote (3) Lichtenstein P, Yip BH, Björk C, Pawitan Y, Cannon TD, Sullivan PF, Hultman CM. Common genetic determinants of schizophrenia and bipolar disorder in Swedish families: a population-based study. Lancet.

Endnote (5) https://www.news-medical.net/health/The-Genetics-of-Mental-Disorder.aspx#

References:

McGuffin P, Owen MJ, Gottesman II. Psychiatric Genetics and Genomics. Oxford: Oxford University Press; 200).

McGuffin P, Rijsdijk F, Andrew M, Sham P, Katz R, Cardno A. The Heritability of Bipolar Affective Disorder and the Genetic Relationship to Unipolar Depression. Arch Gen Psychiatry. 2003;60:497–502.

Klerman & Barrett/Harvard Medical School Clinical Features of Manic Depression" (2:4) https://www.health.harvard.edu/mental-health/bipolar-disorder

Andreasssen, Ole & Hindley, Guy and Frei, Oleksandr and Smeland, Olav. (2023). New insights from the last decade of research in psychiatric genetics: discoveries, challenges and clinical implications. World Psychiatry. 22. 4-24. 10.1002/wps.21034.

Part 5 – The DNA Connection, Epigenetics and Generational Trauma

Endnote (1)
https://truthout.org/articles/intergenerational-trauma-is-a-biological-reality/

Endnote (2)
https://www.theguardian.com/science/2015/aug/21/study-of-holocaust-survivors-finds-trauma-passed-on-to-childrens-genes
https://www.research.va.gov/currents/1016-3.cfm

Endnote (3) Kaiser J. The epigenetics heretic. Science. 2014;343(6169):361-363. doi:10.1126/science.343.6169.361

Endnote (4) Yehuda, Rachel and Daskalakis, Nikolaos and Bierer, Linda and Bader, Heather and Klengel, Torsten and Holsboer, Florian and Binder, Elisabeth. (2015). Holocaust Exposure Induced Intergenerational Effects on FKBP5 Methylation. Biological Psychiatry. 10.1016/j.biopsych.2015.08.005.

Endnote (5) Ido Efrati https://www.haaretz.com/2013-11-26/ty-article/.premium/ashkenazi-geneincreases-schizophrenia/0000017f-e04b-d75c-a7ff-fccfa3e10000

Endnote (6) https://www.cancer.gov/about-cancer/causes-prevention/genetics/brca-genes-hp-pdq#_589, 2023

Endnote (7) https://www.genome.gov/10001356/june-2000-white-house-event#

References:

https://www.nimh.nih.gov/health/publications/looking-at-my-genes

Shamsi, M. B., Firoz, A. S., Imam, S. N., Alzaman, N., and Samman, M. A. (2017). Epigenetics of human diseases and scope in future therapeutics. Journal of Taibah University Medical Sciences, 12(3), 205-211. https://doi.org/10.1016/j.jtumed.2017.04.003

Israeli, American researchers publish work on new genetic risk factor for schizophrenia, bipolar disorder By Judy Siegel-Itzkovich Published: November19, 2013 18:18

Part 6 - Coping, The Stigma

Reference: https://www.bringchange2mind.org/ Glenn Close

Part 6 - Coping, We've Come a Long Way

Endnote (1) https://www.mayoclinic.org/tests-procedures/electroconvulsive-therapy/about/pac-20393894

Endnote (2) https://blog.petrieflom.law.harvard.edu/2020/10/14/why-buck-v-bell-still-matters/#

Endnote (3) https://www.nps.gov/articles/000/rosemary-kennedy-the-eldest-kennedy-daughter.htm#

References:
https://online.csp.edu/resources/article/history-of-mental-illness-treatment/

Payne NA, Prudic J. Electroconvulsive therapy: Part I. A perspective on the evolution and current practice of ECT. J Psychiatr Pract. 2009 Sep;15(5):346-68. doi: 10.1097/01.pra.0000361277.65468.ef. PMID: 19820553; PMCID: PMC3042260.

National Institutes of Health (.gov)
https://pubmed.ncbi.nlm.nih.gov/25311628/

https://www.press.jhu.edu/books/title/12262/three-generations-no-imbeciles, Bell. Buck v Bell
https://edu.lva.virginia.gov/dbva/items/show/227

John Kennedy Presidential Library and Museum

Papers of John F. Kennedy. Presidential Papers. President's Office Files. Legislative Files. Special Message on mental illness and mental retardation, 5 February 1963

Part 6 - Coping, Hope for Genetic Research

Endnote (1)
https://www.nimh.nih.gov/health/publications/looking-at-my-genes

References:
https://pubmed.ncbi.nlm.nih.gov/36640404/

Andreasssen, Ole and Hindley, Guy and Frei, Oleksandr and Smeland, Olav. (2023)

Part 6 - Coping, Hope for Schizophrenia Treatment

Endnote (1)
https://www.theguardian.com/society/2023/jul/30/we-have-hope-for-some-breakthroughs-can-we-change-the-way-we-treat-schizophrenia

Part 6 - Coping, Hope for Technological Advances

Endnote (1) https://swmedical.org/breakthrough-in-using-artificial-intelligence-to-treat-depression/ CDRC), which is part of the O'Donnell Brain Institute University of Texas. University of Texas Southwestern Medical Center's Peter O'Donnell Jr. Brain Institute continues leading at the forefront of neurological breakthroughs. The Center for Depression Research and Clinical Care (CDRC), which is part of the O'Donnell Brain Institute, continues to drive transformative discoveries that are revolutionizing how we diagnose, treat, and prevent mental health and mood disorders. New research from the CDRC will bring more effective depression treatment to patients using artificial intelligence (AI) and brain scans.

Endnote (2) https://woebothealth.com/

Endnote (3) https://www.x2ai.com/uprisehealth

Endnote (4) https://medicalfuturist.com/future-of-psychiatry/

Endnote (5)
https://www.theatlantic.com/magazine/archive/2017/0
7/the-smartphonepsychiatrist/528726/

References:

Farhud DD, Zokaei S. Ethical Issues of Artificial
Intelligence in Medicine and Healthcare. Iran J Public
Health. 2021 Nov;50(11):i-v. doi:
10.18502/ijph.v50i11.7600. PMID: 35223619; PMCID:
PMC8826344.

Sarah Carr (2020) 'AI gone mental': engagement and
ethics in data-driven technology for mental health,
Journal of Mental Health, 29:2, 125-130, DOI:
10.1080/09638237.2020.1714011

Part 6 - Coping, Hope for Mental Health Parity

https://www.samhsa.gov/newsroom/press-
announcements/20220427/hhs-new-mental-health-
substance-use-disorder-benefit-resources/

Part 7 - Traces, Legacy

Endnote (1) https://www.amazon.com/How-Say-
Seniors-Closing-Communication-
ebook/dp/B002GOP9EK/

MARLENE DUNHAM

Acknowledgements

I want to thank my siblings, Claudia, Bruce, Stacey, and Warren for their contributions. All our memories are so different, just like how we were raised and how we have dealt with our past. I feel closer to all of you through this journey. We have never been what you would call a close family, due to age or distance or other reasons. We have never even all been in the same room at the same time. I feel so much more connected now.

There is an old photo I have always held dear to me. I call it The Picture of the Incomplete Family.

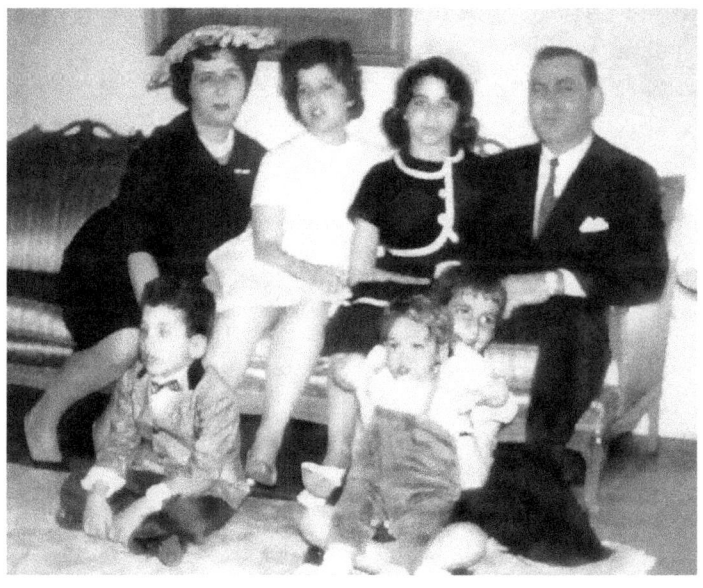

L-R: Joan (Mom), Me (Marlene aka Bunnie), Lorraine, Burt (Dad), Warren (at my feet), Claudia, holding Bruce.
Sometime in 1961.

1. Warren was institutionalized in 1958.

2. Stacey (missing from this photo) wasn't born until 1966.

3. Lorraine committed suicide in 1967.

For about 18 months, between March 23rd of 1966 and October 10th of 1967, all of my family members existed at the same time, however, never in the same room, never in the same place. Stacey never met her brother Warren until 2023, and she certainly doesn't remember her sister Lorraine. In fact, she was never told about Lorraine until she was about seven years old.

I hope I did them all justice by telling their stories within these pages.

Your loving sister,

Bunnie

About the Author

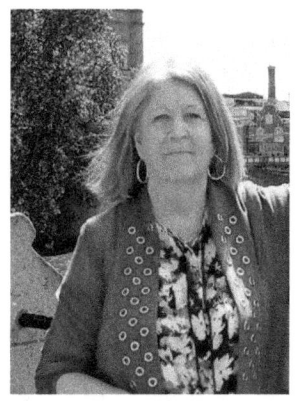

Most of Marlene Dunham's stories are based in the place she was born and raised, New York City. After twenty years working in the city government offices of a Seattle suburb, Marlene has now retired to spend her time writing, traveling, mothering, and grandmothering. Marlene caught the travel bug after discovering her maternal grandfather's place of birth in a tiny southern Italian hill town. There, she met relatives she didn't know existed. As she studied her own genealogy, Marlene became even more fascinated with the intersection of family history and mental health history.

This love of storytelling, family history, and mental health issues was on full display with her contributions to OpenSalon, an online blogsite. Following its demise, Marlene continued writing on her own blog, Dunham's Den.

Marlene Dunham's first non-fiction narrative, *Embracing the Shadows: Navigating a Family's Mental Illness*, tells of her own family's struggles with Bipolar Disease, Schizophrenia, suicide, and acute mental disability. Additionally, this memoir serves to illustrate how our society has progressed in its treatment, diagnosis, and destigmatization of mental illness.